Radiographic Imaging
for Dental Auxiliaries

Radiographic Imaging for Dental Auxiliaries

Third Edition

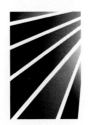

Dale A. Miles, D.D.S., M.S., F.R.C.D.
Professor and Director, Graduate Program
Oral and Maxillofacial Radiology
Indiana University School of Dentistry
Indianapolis, Indiana

Margot L. Van Dis, D.D.S., M.S.
Associate Dean for Education and Student Affairs
Indiana University School of Dentistry
Indianapolis, Indiana

Catherine W. Jensen, R.D.H., B.S., M.H.E.
Director
Southern Illinois Mobile X-Ray Company
Makanda, Illinois

Ann Bruno Ferretti, C.D.A., B.S., M.Ed.
Pensacola, Florida

W.B. SAUNDERS COMPANY
An Imprint of Elsevier Science
Philadelphia   London   New York   St. Louis   Sydney   Toronto

W. B. SAUNDERS COMPANY
An Imprint of Elsevier Science
The Curtis Center
Independence Square West
Philadelphia, PA 19106

Library of Congress Cataloging-in-Publication Data

Radiographic imaging for dental auxiliaries / Dale A. Miles . . . [et al.].—3rd ed.

p.   cm.

Includes index.

ISBN 0–7216–8016–X

1. Teeth—Radiography.   2. Dental auxiliary personnel.   I. Miles, Dale A.

RK309.R28 1999   617.6′07572—dc21

DNLM/DLC   98–27545

RADIOGRAPHIC IMAGING FOR DENTAL AUXILIARIES   ISBN 0–7216–8016–X

Printed in the United States of America.

Last digit is the print number: 9   8   7   6   5   4

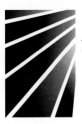

Preface

It has been 10 years since the first edition of this book was published. I am thankful for the many comments from instructors of oral and maxillofacial radiology who took the time to read the text so carefully and offer suggestions for improvement. Most of the changes have been made, and the book continues to improve. I imagine that the students who used this book all practice safe x-ray management and produce excellent diagnostic radiographs in the practices where they work. For this accomplishment, their employers and their patients must be grateful. As for my fellow authors and myself, it makes us proud to have made this positive contribution to dental practice and to successful training of dental hygienists and dental assistants in North America.

To the instructors who have used this textbook in the past, I think that you will find the up-to-date, timely chapters, *Digital Imaging* and *Implant Imaging*, explaining charge-coupled devices (CCDs) and photostimulable phosphors extremely useful in training your students for these newer modalities. I believe that this information, explained in a clear and precise way, will help you to prepare your students for the ever-changing science and art of dental imaging.

To the instructors who have not used our textbook in the past to teach the basic principles of dental imaging, I'd like you to take another look at the textbook you're using now by comparison. I think that the third edition of *Radiographic Imaging for Dental Auxiliaries* is the most complete and the most contemporary textbook available for your students. I hope that you will consider complementing your own teaching materials with this book. I think that your students will appreciate the useful, well-illustrated, and well-organized information it contains.

To the students, we hope that we have provided one of the best educational aids you will require to master the art and science of dentomaxillofacial radiology. Good luck to you all!

DAM
MLVD
CWJ
ABF

Acknowledgments

This third edition would not have been possible without the efforts of the following people: Ms. Julie LeHunt, Administrative Secretary, Department of Oral Surgery, Medicine, and Pathology; Mr. Mike Halloran, photographer extraordinaire and Mr. Mark Dirlam, graphic artist, Department of Dental Art and Illustrations at Indiana University School of Dentistry.

I also wish to thank Ms. Shirley Kuhn, Associate Editor, Health-Related Professions; her assistant, Ms. Katherine Macciocca; and Ms. Michaelina Lombardi, developmental editor, and her husband, Mr. H. R. Lombardi, for their persistence in keeping us moving forward with the myriad details that make a book successful.

DAM
MLVD
CWJ
ABF

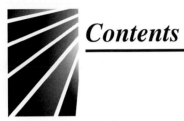

Contents

Chapter 11

Normal Anatomy and Film Mounting 211

Chapter 12

Interpretation: Normal Versus Abnormal and Common Radiographic Presentation of Lesions 231

Chapter 13

Radiation Biology and Protection 281

Chapter 1

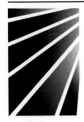

Intraoral Radiographic Technique

BEFORE YOU BEGIN

X radiation, what you will be using to produce radiographs (x-ray films), is biologically damaging. Any exposure, no matter how insignificant it may seem, has the potential to damage living tissue—yours or your patient's. You need to begin your radiologic education by practicing techniques and skills and by acquiring habits that will protect both you and your patient. The beginning of this chapter gives you enough practical guidelines to complete laboratory exercises safely on a radiographic phantom or skull. For those who begin practice on patients early, a summary of patient protection procedures is also included. An in-depth discussion of radiation biology, protection procedures, and legal aspects is presented in Chapter 13.

Practical Guidelines

1. **Never do anything to your patient that you would not like to have done to you.**
2. **It is easier to do it right the first time than to explain why you did it wrong.**

These basic rules are the foundation for most of the safety and protection procedures.

Before you set foot in a radiographic operatory, you should be familiar with the equipment. To use the equipment properly, you need to be able to select "exposure settings" correctly. These exposure settings may vary for different units. Your instructor will have determined the correct exposure settings in advance; your responsibility is to know the correct settings and how to change the settings if they are incorrect. Federal guidelines state that a chart showing settings for time (seconds or impulses), kilovolt peak (kVp), and milliamperage (mA) for commonly used techniques should be posted close to the control panel of each x-ray unit. Check with your instructor about the location of this chart (Fig. 1–1).

Operator Protection

One of your additional responsibilities is to learn and practice some basic rules of *operator protection* relating to your laboratory practice.

1. **Never** stand in the direct line of the primary beam (the open end of the cylinder, where the radiation exits the unit). It is best to stand behind a lead barrier (Fig. 1–2). If you cannot place an acceptable barrier between you and the beam, stand at right angles to the beam (Fig. 1–3).

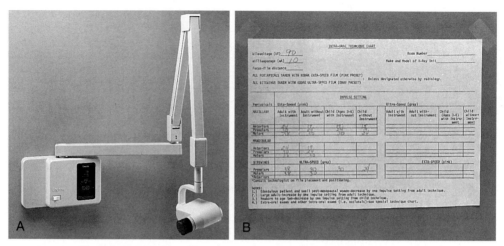

Figure 1–1. A, Radiographic equipment. B, Accompanying exposure setting chart.

2. **Never** hold the film in a patient's mouth or in any radiographic training phantom. If the patient cannot hold the film without help, use alternative placement methods.
3. **Never** stand closer than 6 feet to the x-ray unit during an exposure.
4. **Never** use equipment that is faulty or that you suspect is faulty. For example, if the x-ray tubehead drifts (moves) after it is positioned, the unit should be repaired before further use. If noises, sparks, or smoke comes from the unit during an exposure, the unit should not be used until repaired. *Anything out of the ordinary should be reported to the appropriate person before the equipment is used again.*

Patient Protection

Radiographic practice on clinical patients should not begin until a reasonable level of competency is achieved in a closely supervised laboratory environment. Principles of *patient protection* must be understood prior to exposing patients to x radiation.

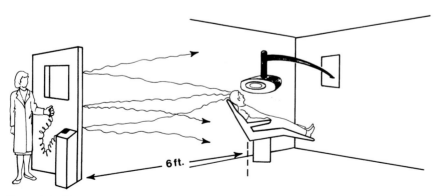

Figure 1–2. The operator stands behind a protective lead-walled barrier. The patient is visible to the operator throughout the procedure.

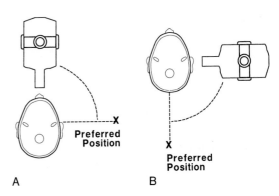

Figure 1–3. *A,* The X shows the preferred position for the operator during the x-ray exposure of an anterior film. The region between the tubehead and the X is also considered "safe." *B,* The preferred position for a posterior film exposure.

1. Radiographs should never be made on a patient unless they offer a *benefit* to the patient that *outweighs the risk* of the radiation exposure.
2. Each patient should be shielded as much as possible. Protection should include a **leaded apron** and a **leaded thyroid shield.**
3. **Long "cone" paralleling technique** for intraoral films is recommended by the American Dental Association and by the American Academy of Oral and Maxillofacial Radiology unless circumstances or anatomy dictate the use of other techniques. The paralleling technique not only produces a better radiograph with less distortion and greater accuracy, but also significantly reduces patient radiation dose.
4. **Proper exposure and processing techniques** should be employed to produce the most diagnostically useful films. *Minimizing retakes necessitated by improper exposure or processing may be the single most effective method for reducing radiation exposure to patients.*

Patient and Operator Protection

1. *Always review the patient's medical history* for the possibility of infectious disease, for medical problems that may complicate radiography, and, in the case of females of childbearing years, for pregnancy.
   A policy regarding pregnant patients should be established and strictly followed. Many experts recommend that elective radiographic procedures be postponed until the patient is no longer pregnant.
2. *Always wear clean gloves* when performing radiographic procedures. The universal precautions of the Centers for Disease Control and Prevention (CDC) should be followed during radiographic procedures for all patients. Some guidelines appear at the end of this chapter.

INTRAORAL RADIOGRAPHIC TECHNIQUES

Radiographs are two-dimensional images of three-dimensional objects. The objects that are radiographed have *length* and *width* and *depth,* yet the image on the radiographic film is a representation that has only length and width. The depth, or thickness, of the object cannot be determined on the film. The images produced on a radiographic film represent a number of the patient's anatomic structures superimposed over each other. The films afford the clinician an opportunity to "look inside" and "see" internal structures as if they were transparent (Fig. 1–4).

The patient's anatomic structures need to be reconstructed in the mind's eye. Simply looking at the image may not tell the viewer whether structures are facial (to the outside of the dental arch) or lingual (to the inside of the arch).

Intraoral Film Types

Dental radiographs may be intraoral or extraoral. *Intraoral* radiographs are made by placing the x-ray film inside the mouth and projecting x radiation from a source outside the face, through the anatomic structures of interest (the object), and onto the film. *Extraoral* radiographs, discussed in a later chapter, are made by placing the film outside the oral cavity.

There are three types of intraoral radiographs: (1) periapical, (2) bitewing, and (3) occlusal. Periapical and bitewing radiographs are the most commonly used intraoral projections in dentistry (Figs. 1–5 through 1–7).

Periapical radiographs record images of the teeth (outlines, positions, dimensions) as well as supporting structures such as trabecular bone, lamina dura, and periodontal membrane space. Each film usually contains an image of a group of teeth in one area of the arch at a time. Periapical films are used to interpret normal anatomy and pathology in the root area and in the surrounding bony structures. It is critical to obtain an image that includes the *entire length of the teeth of interest plus 3–4 mm of supporting tissue beyond the root apex* (Fig. 1–8).

Bitewing radiographs record images of the *crowns* and *interproximal* regions of maxillary and mandibular teeth on the same film (Figs. 1–9 and 1–10). Film placement in this technique generally produces a more anatomically and dimensionally accurate image than that seen in a periapical view. However, the image is limited to the coronal one-third of the teeth and related structures. This type of radiograph is used to reveal interproximal or recurrent carious lesions (cavities), overhanging restorations, calculus, crestal bone levels, internal pulpal pathology,

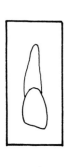

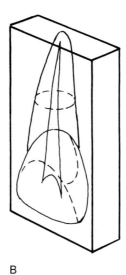

Figure 1–4. A, Two-dimensional radiograph. *B,* Three-dimensional object or structure that was radiographed. We "see" internal structures; in reality, these structures are superimposed over one another, each stopping a different number of x rays.

A   B

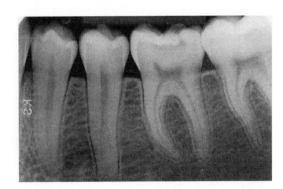

Figure 1–5. Periapical radiograph of the mandibular left premolar region.

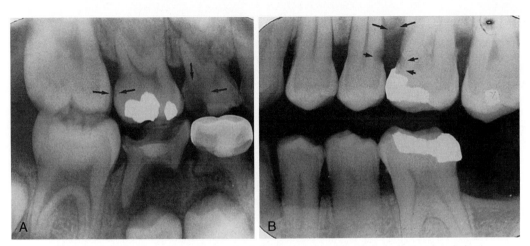

Figure 1–6. *A,* Bitewing radiograph of a mixed dentition, used to detect interproximal carious lesions *(arrows). B,* Adult bitewing radiograph demonstrating both root caries *(small arrows)* and bone loss *(large arrows).*

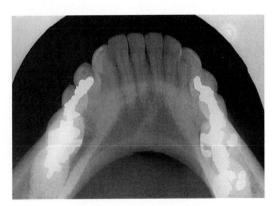

Figure 1–7. Typical mandibular occlusal radiograph (see Chapter 6 on accessory techniques).

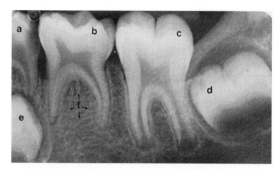

Figure 1–8. Periapical radiograph of a 7- to 8-year-old child, showing the erupted primary and the developing permanent teeth in the mandibular left quadrant: *a*, primary first molar; *b*, primary second molar; *c*, permanent first molar; *d*, developing permanent second molar; *e*, developing permanent first bicuspid; *f*, region of the permanent second bicuspid that failed to develop.

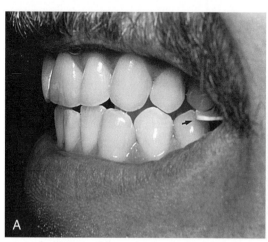

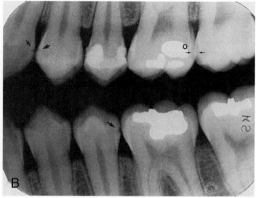

Figure 1–9. *A*, This clinical photograph shows the difficulty in visualizing the film placement when the patient has closed on the "bite tab," a cardboard loop used to hold the film. If the film is centered in the holder, then the tab *(black arrow)* should be centered at the second premolar/first molar contact, as illustrated. *B*, This premolar bitewing view shows the correct positioning of the teeth. All contacts between the teeth are "open," and the distal half of each canine is included on the film. Carious lesions are then visible with no overlap between the enamel of adjacent teeth *(arrows)*. Overlap is, however, shown between the maxillary first and second molars *(o)*.

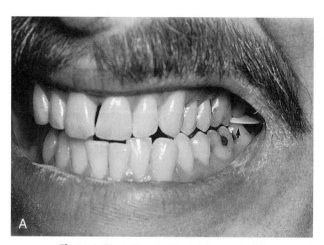

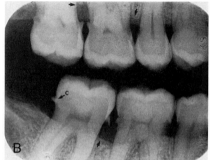

Figure 1–10. *A*, This is the correct position of the bite tab between the maxillary and mandibular second molars *(arrow)*. This placement will ensure "open" contacts in the *molar* region. *B*, The resultant molar bitewing views, showing bone loss *(arrows)* and interproximal calculus, seen as white "spikes" between the teeth in this view *(c)*.

and occlusal relationships. Bitewing films offer a diagnostic aid for detecting incipient (enamel) carious lesions not detectable by any other clinical method. Bitewing radiographs also provide the most accurate assessment of interproximal alveolar crestal bone height. The use of bitewings for incipient cavity detection will become even more important as the use of sealants and other preventive materials increases.

Occlusal radiographs record images of an entire arch on one film. There are several useful projections for occlusal radiographs (Figs. 1–11 and 1–12). The technique, purpose, and interpretation of occlusal films are discussed in more detail in Chapter 6.

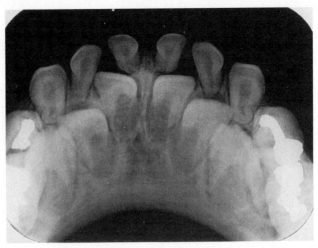

Figure 1–11. Mandibular occlusal radiograph of the primary dentition of a child about 4 years old.

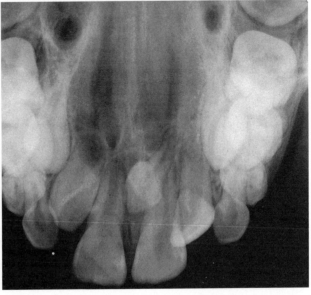

Figure 1–12. Maxillary occlusal radiograph of the same child as in Figure 1–11. Note the extra toothlike structure between the central incisors. This is called a "mesiodens." (See also Chapter 12.)

TYPES OF RADIOGRAPHIC SURVEYS:
BWS, CMRS (FMX)

Two common dental radiographic surveys are the *bitewing survey (BWS)* and the *complete mouth radiographic survey (CMRS)* or *full mouth x-ray series (FMX)*. The BWS normally consists of two or four posterior films with molars grouped together and premolars grouped together. Both left and right sides of the patient's mouth are radiographed (Figs. 1–13 and 1–14).

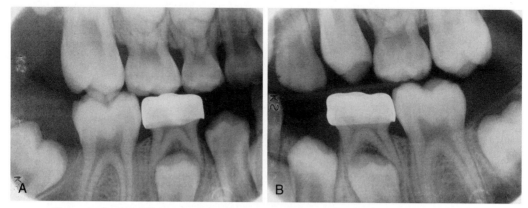

Figure 1–13. Left *(A)* and right *(B)* bitewing radiographs of a child. Only two bitewing films are required.

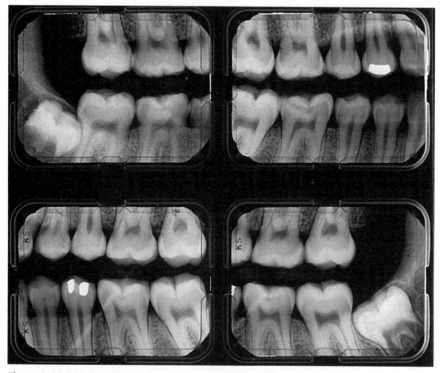

Figure 1–14. Left *(bottom)* and right *(top)* bitewing radiographs of an adult. Four bitewing films are needed to ensure that all contacts are "open."

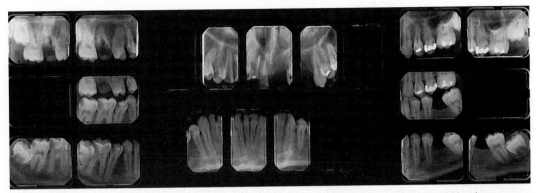

Figure 1–15. Typical complete mouth radiographic series, showing selected periapical and bitewing films.

The CMRS, or FMX, is composed of a number of periapical radiographs. This survey may or may not include bitewings, but it must include *every tooth, every apex, every contact area, 3–4 mm of supporting structure periapically, and all toothbearing areas* (even though the patient may be edentulous) *at least once somewhere on the survey.* To obtain radiographic images of all of these structures, an operator may take as few as 10 or as many as 18 periapical films, plus whichever bitewing films are indicated. The number and size of film to use in a CMRS depend upon the number of teeth present, the size of the oral cavity, the anatomic structures within the mouth, the age of the patient, the specific technique, and the level of patient cooperation (Fig. 1–15).

Complete mouth radiographic surveys may be performed using either a paralleling or a bisecting-angle technique. The American Dental Association and the American Academy of Oral and Maxillofacial Radiology recommend the use of the *paralleling technique* for routine periapical exposures; in accordance with these recommendations, the remainder of this book considers paralleling as the standard technique. Paralleling is also the most appropriate technique for digital image acquisition using charge-coupled devices (CCDs). This is discussed more fully in Chapter 10. Nevertheless, the bisecting-angle technique remains a valuable accessory technique and, as such, has been included in Chapter 6.

Film Sizes for CMRS

X-ray film is the medium used to record anatomic images. Five commonly used sizes are shown in Figure 1–16. Complete mouth radiographic surveys for adults normally use film sizes no. 1 and no. 2. Adult bitewing surveys normally use no. 2 size film. Smaller film, size no. 0, may be used for children less than 3 years old. Note that anterior films are placed with the longest dimension vertically, and posterior films are placed horizontally (Fig. 1–17).

The Need for Each Film Type

A common misconception among beginning radiography students is that areas that have no teeth (edentulous areas) do not need to be radiographed. The purpose of radiographing edentulous regions is to aid in diagnosing problems that cannot

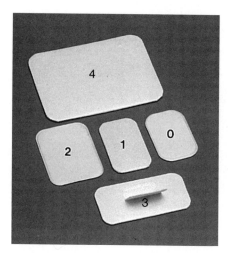

Figure 1–16. Photograph of the five sizes of intraoral radiographic films. Film size no. 0 is used for children with primary dentition; no. 1 is used for mixed dentition radiographs and, in many cases, for anterior views in adult dentition; no. 2 is used for both vertical and horizontal positions, mainly in adult dentition; no. 3 is used for occlusal radiographs; no. 4 is a longer version of the no. 2 size film and is used for interproximal bitewing radiographs.

be seen clinically. Such problems may include more than just the tooth-related ones. The appearance of supporting structures, such as bone and soft tissues, may reflect health or disease. Changes in trabecular pattern, the presence or absence of structures, and other radiographic alterations may provide information regarding a patient's health status. Therefore, periapical films of areas where teeth are not clinically present should also be included in the CMRS or FMX if the dentist has so prescribed.

The need for bitewing radiographs is different. Bitewings are needed only in areas where teeth have interproximal contact with other teeth, obstructing a clinical view of the mesial and distal surfaces. The primary use of bitewing radiographs is to detect interproximal carious lesions (recall Figs. 1–6 and 1–9). If interproximal

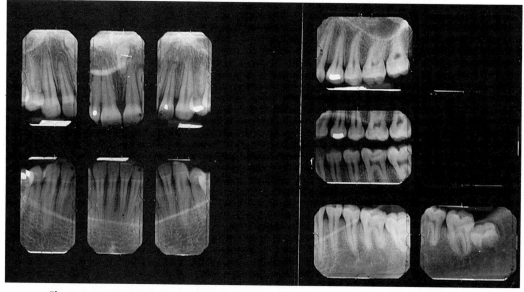

Figure 1–17. Photograph of six anterior and four posterior films. The anterior views are size no. 1. All are in the vertical position. The molar views are size no. 2, used in a horizontal position. The maxillary molar periapical view and the molar bitewing view were not necessary, and two blank, processed (black) films are placed in the mount to block extraneous light.

spaces can be examined clinically, there may be no need for a particular bitewing radiograph.

Because in a facial-to-lingual dimension the anterior teeth are thinner than the posterior teeth, it may be much easier to see the interproximal spaces with direct vision and transillumination. These procedures eliminate the need for anterior bitewings in most cases.

INTRAORAL RADIOGRAPHY—BASIC PRINCIPLES

Paralleling Periapical Technique

The paralleling periapical technique is employed in dental radiography to minimize shape distortion of the radiographic image and to reduce x radiation dose to the patient's head and neck. The geometric principle of this technique is to place the film parallel to the long axes of the teeth to be radiographed while aiming the central x ray (central ray, CR, or x-ray beam), perpendicular to both. Certain basic principles must be understood when periapical intraoral radiographic techniques are practiced:

1. Anatomic considerations.
2. X-ray beam angulation.
3. Point of entry.
4. Film packet placement.

Anatomic Considerations

Location of Long Axes of the Teeth. Most root apices in the maxilla tilt inward toward the palate. The flatter or more shallow the palatal vault of the maxilla is, the greater the tendency for the apices to tilt inward. The crowns of the six anterior teeth usually tilt outward (Fig. 1–18).

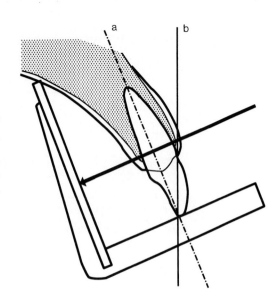

Figure 1–18. Schematic drawing of tilting of maxillary anterior teeth. The film parallels the long axis *(dotted line a)*; however, the operator sees only the crowns, and the inclination of the crown seems more vertically oriented *(solid line b)*.

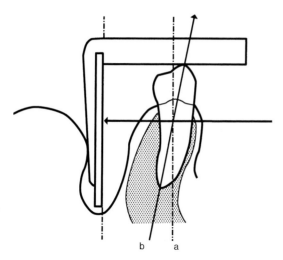

Figure 1–19. The long axis *(solid line b)* of this bicuspid is less vertical than one would expect from looking at the teeth clinically *(dotted line a)*.

The mandibular premolars are more nearly vertical (Fig. 1–19). Mandibular molars tilt inward slightly. Whereas the crowns of the teeth appear to tilt one way, the entire structure actually tilts another; you cannot assume that roots are perfectly vertical just because the crowns appear to be so.

This concept is important because the film is placed parallel to the long axis of the *whole tooth* in the paralleling technique, not just parallel to the crown. In addition, anatomic structures such as the palate or the floor of the mouth may influence the extent to which the film can parallel the long axes of the teeth. The anatomy of a patient's mouth may dictate the use of an alternative technique or modification of the paralleling principle.

Location of the Apices and Respective Head Positions. The apical region of the maxillary teeth is located on an imaginary line drawn from the ala of the nose to the tragus of the ear (Fig. 1–20). It may be helpful to have the ala-tragus line

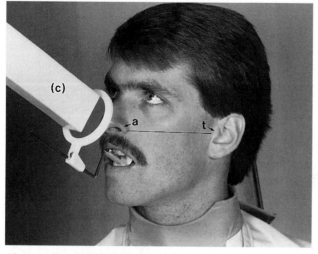

Figure 1–20. Ala-tragus line. The ala *(a)* is the side of the nose. The tragus is labeled *t*. This line closely parallels the tips of the maxillary teeth from canine to third molar; it is easier to visualize than the occlusal plane when the patient has closed. Here we have pictured a typical rectangular "cone" or "cylinder," labeled *(c)*.

parallel to the floor when radiographing maxillary teeth. This makes the maxillary occlusal plane parallel to the floor also. The correct head position is your starting point.

The paralleling technique requires the use of a film-holding device. Many of the film-holding devices have an extraoral marker of some sort, usually a locator ring to help you position the x-ray tube exactly over the film (Fig. 1–21). When using these devices, you may place the patient in almost any position you choose and still produce quality radiographs. The most important point to remember is to place the patient in a position that will make the procedure successful and the patient comfortable.

X-Ray Beam Angulation: Vertical and Horizontal

Vertical Angulation. The x-ray tube has two directional positions that must be adjusted during an exposure. The *vertical angulation* is the movement of the tubehead up and down, similar to someone nodding his or her head "yes." If the x-ray tubehead is pointing down, the angulation is positive. If the x-ray tubehead is pointing up, the angulation is negative. Many x-ray units have dials on the arms that indicate the positive or negative angulation by degrees. Using the floor as a reference, the tubehead would be parallel to it at zero degrees (0°). If the tubehead were pointing straight down, the vertical angulation would be positive 90 degrees (+90°); if the tubehead were pointing straight upward, the vertical angulation would be negative 90 degrees (−90°). This concept is illustrated in Figure 1–22. The vertical angle of the x-ray beam must be perpendicular both to the film and to the long axes of the teeth in the paralleling technique.

Horizontal Angulation. The *horizontal angulation* is the position of the x-ray tube in the same direction as the horizon. Horizontal angulation movement may be compared to someone shaking his or her head "no." The horizontal angles

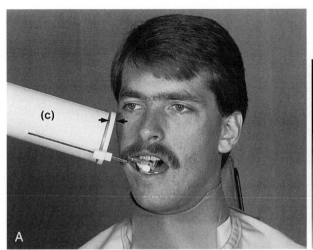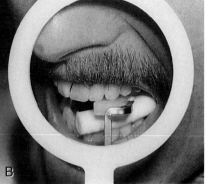

Figure 1–21. *A,* The locator ring *(arrows)* is attached to a metal rod, which in turn holds the film. The cylinder *(c)* is aligned precisely with the locator ring and the metal rod in both horizontal and vertical directions. *B,* The tooth of interest—the cuspid—is centered in the ring.

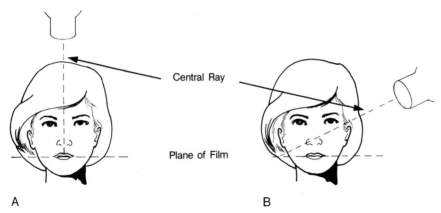

Figure 1–22. *A,* Positive 90 degrees (+90°). *B,* Positive vertical angulation.

rotate around the patient's head 360 degrees, as if the head were the center of a circle. Imagine someone standing behind a tree. If you look directly at the front of the tree, you cannot see any part of the person behind it. If you move in a wide circle around the tree, you will begin to see the person behind the tree because you are changing the horizontal angle of your vision. Keep this example in mind when you think of horizontal angulation. The horizontal angulation of the x-ray beam should be directed through the contacts of the teeth, as perpendicular to the horizontal plane of the film as possible (Fig. 1–23).

Point of Entry

The point of entry of the x-ray beam should be directed through the center of the region being radiographed. The objective is to completely cover the film with the beam of radiation. If this is not done, a "cone-cut," or partial, image, will be seen in the resultant film (Fig. 1–24). The use of film-holding devices that have extraoral markers can reduce the problem with cone-cut images. A detailed discussion of errors such as these comes later.

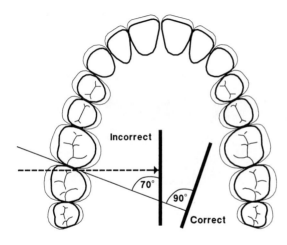

Figure 1–23. In this diagram the parallel x rays pass precisely through the contact areas of the teeth, because the tubehead cylinder is angled at 90 degrees to the film plane. If the film is angled less than 90 degrees to the x rays, overlap of the enamel areas will occur (see Chapter 5 for a more thorough explanation of horizontal angulation errors).

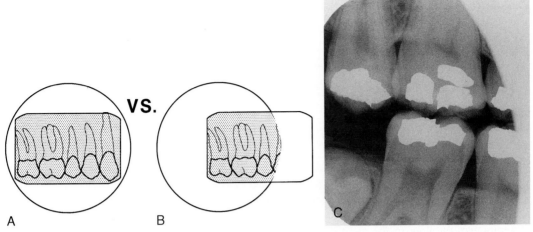

Figure 1–24. *A,* This diagram demonstrates the correct position of the cylinder over the area to be radiographed. *B,* Cone positioned too far distally, so that the anterior portion of the film receives no exposure. *C,* The resultant radiographic image.

Film Packet Placement

Vertical Placement

Maxillary Arch. The film should be placed so that it parallels the long axis of the tooth. This is accomplished by placing the film toward the midline of the palate. If the film packet is placed directly against the lingual side of the teeth, one of three things will happen:

1. The film will not be parallel to the long axes of the teeth, producing an image that is foreshortened, looking as if it were squashed (Fig. 1–25).
2. The film will not be high enough in the palate to capture the image of the apices, resulting in an image with a large margin at the occlusal or incisal edge and with the apices cut off (Fig. 1–26).
3. The film will bend beyond the end of the biteblock, producing a distorted image that looks as if the top of it just slid off the film (Fig. 1–27).

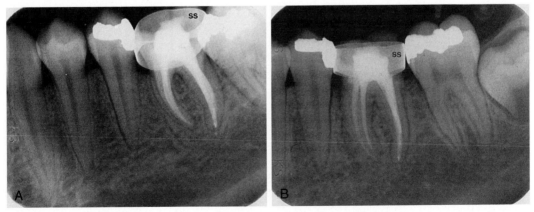

Figure 1–25. *A,* The radiographic image that results if the film is not parallel to long axes of teeth. *B,* The correct image; note that the stainless steel crown *(ss)* appears more anatomically correct than the one in *A.*

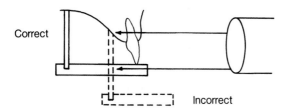

Figure 1–26. Film contacts palate, but the instrument is *not* contacting teeth of interest. The apices will *not* be recorded and, in the resultant image, there will be a large black area below the occlusal edges of the teeth providing no useful information (see Fig. 1–28).

The anatomy of the palate and the placement of the biteblock will determine the final vertical angle of the x-ray beam as the patient closes on the biteblock.

Mandibular Arch. The mandible has a much different shape than the maxilla. The floor of the mouth is occupied by musculature, including the tongue. Because it is muscular, the floor of the mouth can be flexible or rigid. When tensed, it is almost as firm as the hard palate. The apices of the mandibular teeth do not tilt as far inward as those of the maxillary arch, and hence the film packet should not tilt as much. In order to keep the film packet from tilting, the film must be placed low down into the floor of the mouth, actually displacing the tissue. If the patient tenses the muscles of the floor of the mouth, the procedure may be painful, especially if the film is placed too close to the mylohyoid ridge, and the patient may not fully close on the biteblock.

It is rare that anyone has such a shallow floor of the mouth that the films will not fit. More often the projection is unsuccessful because the patient is apprehensive or sensitive, or both, and tenses the muscles of the floor of the mouth. *It is imperative that the floor of the mouth stay relaxed.* One method of film placement is to angle the lower film edge *away* from teeth initially, and then bring the biteblock into contact with incisal edges. Ask the patient to close slowly, and rotate the instrument upward as the patient closes, bringing the film more parallel to the teeth. The

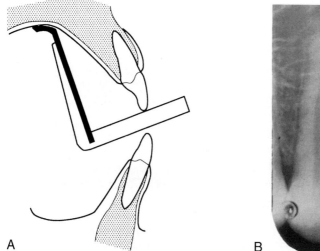

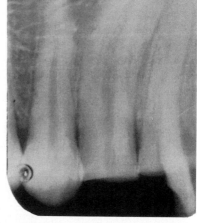

A   B

Figure 1–27. *A,* Diagram of film bending as it contacts the palate. *B,* The resultant image. Note that only the apical areas are blurred and distorted unlike the case of a motion artifact, in which the whole image is blurred.

patient's floor of the mouth will stay more relaxed, and the procedure will be more comfortable.

The second problem is managing the patient's tongue, which may seem to have a mind of its own. Asking the patient to do something with the tongue usually makes the tongue more active and difficult to work around; relaxation techniques and psychology work better. The tongue acts as a physical barrier in the center of the mouth. Obviously, the mandibular films will have to be placed *between* the tongue and the lingual side of the teeth.

Common problems associated with mandibular film placement are as follows:

1. The film may be placed *too close to the lingual side* of the teeth (either because the tongue pushed it there or the operator placed it there). This placement may cause one of two problems:
   a. The film may not be parallel with the long axes of the teeth because of the inclined plane of the lingual alveolar ridge, resulting in a foreshortened image.
   b. The film may not reach into the floor of the mouth, resulting in an image with a wide black area above the crowns and apices that are "cut off" (Fig. 1–28).
2. The tongue may be trapped under the bottom edge of the film packet, resulting in any of the following three problems:
   a. The film may bend because of the pressure of the tongue, producing a blurred, unsharp image.
   b. The film may not reach the floor of the mouth, producing a widely distorted occlusal image, with the apices "cut off."
   c. The film may have proper position and angulation, but the image of the tongue may appear on the processed film. As long as this image can be identified as the soft-tissue shadow of the tongue and as long as the teeth are clearly represented, this technique error is minor (Fig. 1–29).

The following technique will help you to avoid the previously discussed problems: Position the packet in the desired posterior region, but do not force the film

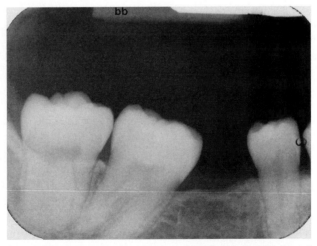

Figure 1–28. This type of image occurs in either the maxillary or the mandibular arch, where patient anatomy prevents imaging of the apices of the teeth of interest. The biteblock *(bb)* can be seen far above the teeth in this mandibular view.

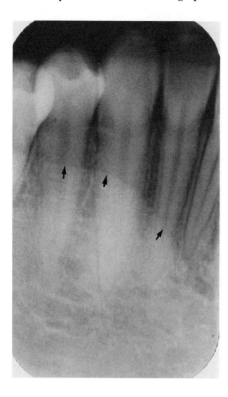

Figure 1–29. Image of the soft tissue of the tongue is seen here *(arrows)* but does not interfere significantly with interpretation.

into the floor of the mouth. A variety of film placement techniques work well for different people under different circumstances. These suggestions will increase the likelihood of success with mandibular films.

Tilt the film away from the mylohyoid ridge as you are placing it in the mouth, making an inverted "V," or tent, with the biteblock over the occlusal surfaces. Place your index finger in the patient's mouth so that it is between the film packet and the mylohyoid ridge. When you rock or slide the film into position on the floor of the mouth, your finger will keep you from scraping the alveolar mucosa with the edge of the film packet. The film can then be positioned for proper mesial/distal placement and correct horizontal angulation.

These simple but important technique tips may mean the difference between success and failure with some patients.

Horizontal Placement: Maxillary or Mandibular. The horizontal placement of the film packet is the critical factor in avoiding overlapped images owing to the incorrect horizontal angulation and in avoiding loss of visualization of anatomic structures owing to incorrect anterior-posterior placement of the film. The placement of the film packet (by virtue of the placement of the biteblock) will determine correct horizontal angulation and correct anterior-posterior film placement at the same time.

The film must be placed in a well-defined anterior-posterior position (the distance forward or backward in the mouth) to afford a view of the correct anatomy. These guidelines are described in detail later in this chapter under the heading "Anatomic Structures in Each Film."

The horizontal angle is determined by selecting a contact point through which to direct the x-ray beam (sometimes called the *direction of the central ray*). Figure 1–30 illustrates examples of this principle. Correct positioning is crucial to obtaining an "open contact" and clear view of the interproximal areas of interest.

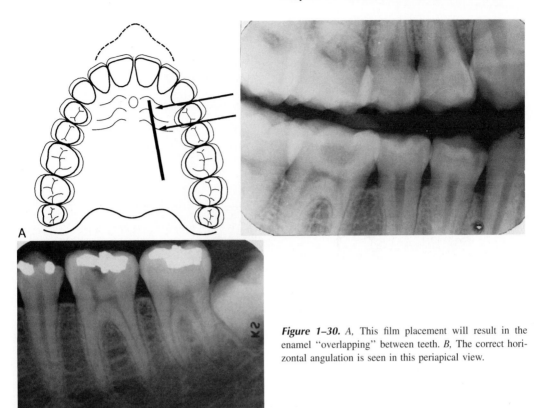

Figure 1–30. *A,* This film placement will result in the enamel "overlapping" between teeth. *B,* The correct horizontal angulation is seen in this periapical view.

Bitewing or Interproximal Techniques

Horizontal Placement. Correct angulation in the horizontal placement of the film packet for a bitewing radiograph is crucial to the diagnostic value of the film. Even a slight amount of overlap may lead to a misdiagnosis (Fig. 1–31). The goal is to obtain bitewings with *no overlapping*. Extra films may be required owing to anatomic deviations and rotated or misaligned teeth.

Vertical Placement. Whether you are using a cardboard tab or a film-holding instrument, it is important that the film not be forced into an inaccurate position by the maxillary teeth. The operator can avoid this problem by simply tilting the top of the film packet lingually as the patient closes. The film should then move into the proper vertical position as the teeth occlude with the tab or the biteblock.

Anterior-Posterior Placement. A good basic setup on molar films is to place the biteblock over the second molar. This technique ensures room on the film for both the first and third molars or molar space. However, as you will see in premolar films, precise anterior-posterior placement is absolutely critical—not only to get the appropriate anatomic structures, but also to avoid placement errors resulting from a patient's individual anatomic variation.

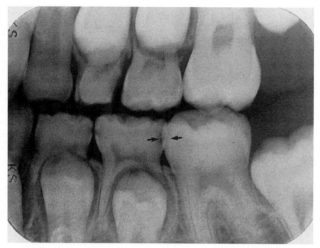

Figure 1–31. Overlap *(arrows)* between the mandibular primary second molar and permanent first molar obscures detection of the carious lesion on the molar.

One final thought about the importance of open contacts on bitewings: Because the primary purpose of a bitewing is to obtain a clear view of the contact areas and the interproximal spaces, overlapping on a bitewing is a critical error. Overlapped images on periapical films are technical errors, but they are not as serious as those on bitewing films because the purpose of a periapical film is to image the periapical areas.

PARALLELING TECHNIQUE

Paralleling Instruments—Film-Holding Devices

Paralleling techniques require the use of film-holding devices. One of the most commonly used types is the RINN XCP instrument* (extension cone paralleling). The technique descriptions that follow are for use with the RINN XCP technique, but the basic principles of placement and paralleling are similar no matter which film-holding device is used.

Advantages. The extraoral marker or locator ring on the film holder makes it easier to set the position of the cylinder without a risk of cone-cut images, a definite advantage over using tabs or film holders without rings (recall Fig. 1–21). The bar or rod connecting the biteblock with the ring can be compared with the line between the contacts to help determine horizontal angulation. Most film holders also keep the film from bending and make it more stable, holding it in position. The only disadvantage to using a film holder is the possibility of patient discomfort. If you correctly assemble the XCP instrument and look through the ring, the biteblock and the film should be centered in the ring (Fig. 1–32).

*RINN XCP instrument, Dentsply RINN Corporation, Elgin, IL.

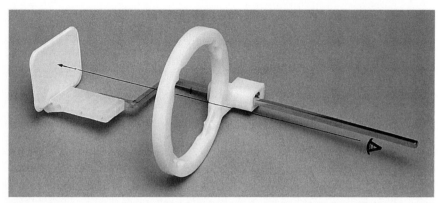

Figure 1–32. Correctly assembled positioning instrument, with film in biteblock centered in the ring.

Consequently, no matter where you position the film in the mouth, it will be centered in the x-ray beam. This technique aids proper placement of the tubehead and the open-ended cylinder, but proper film placement is still required. The open-ended cylinder is placed directly against the ring. Such placement helps ensure that (1) the beam will always be perpendicular to the film, and (2) the x-ray beam will be centered over the entire film packet.

Film Packet Placement. The following pages outline the techniques for periapical and bitewing radiography using paralleling principles and a conventional film-holding device. Correct film placement will be illustrated for each view.

Anatomic Structures in Each Film

A typical complete mouth radiographic survey using the paralleling technique consists of 14 to 16 periapical projections and four bitewing projections (Fig. 1–33). Each film must be placed so that it covers the appropriate anatomic structures, as described in the following section.

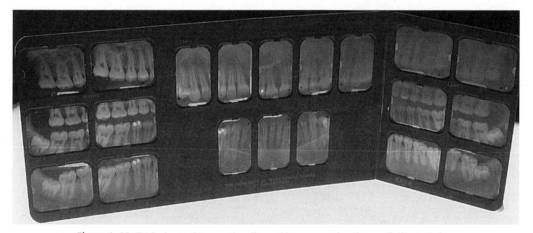

Figure 1–33. Typical complete mouth radiographic survey using the paralleling technique.

PARALLELING TECHNIQUE

Maxillary Central Incisor Region

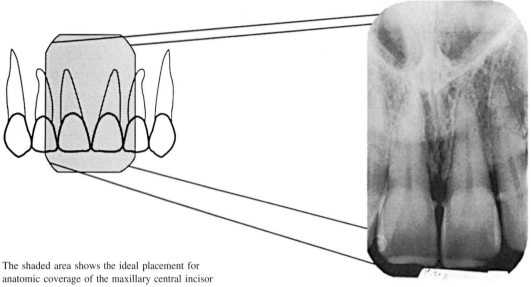

The shaded area shows the ideal placement for anatomic coverage of the maxillary central incisor region.

In this view the maxillary central incisors are centered on the biteblock (see also diagram on facing page). If you use a size no. 2 film, the apices and crowns of all four incisors should be visible on the radiograph. Slightly less anatomic coverage is demonstrated with the size no. 1 film used here.

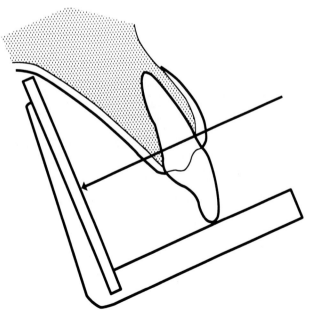

The plastic biteblock contacts the palate and the teeth of interest and is parallel to the long axis of the tooth. The film should never be placed against the teeth; rather, as much of the biteblock as possible should be used to place the film near the center of the palate. The central ray is directed perpendicular (at 90 degrees) to the film plane.

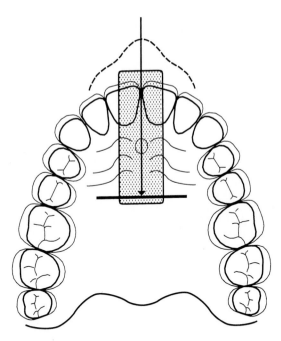

The diagram shows that the central incisors are centered, and the film is positioned well into the oral cavity.

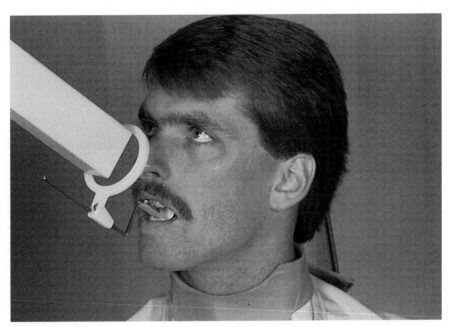

Final positioning of film and instrument. The patient is asked to close slowly and firmly on the biteblock. Note that here a rectangular "cylinder" is shown and that the lower edge of the cylinder parallels the metallic indicating rod. The cylinder is brought to within ½ inch or less from the plastic ring. The exposure is made. Operators often struggle with making the last little tube adjustments. Often it is easier to move the patient's face a little bit than to struggle with the tubehead and position-indicating device.

PARALLELING TECHNIQUE

Maxillary Lateral Incisor Region

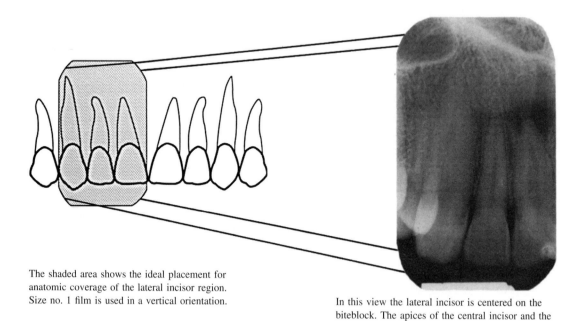

The shaded area shows the ideal placement for anatomic coverage of the lateral incisor region. Size no. 1 film is used in a vertical orientation.

In this view the lateral incisor is centered on the biteblock. The apices of the central incisor and the cuspid area are also visible.

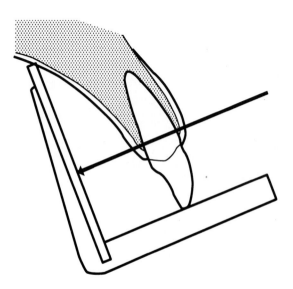

This diagram and the one on the facing page show the positioning of the film near the center of the palate. The central ray is directed perpendicular to the film plane.

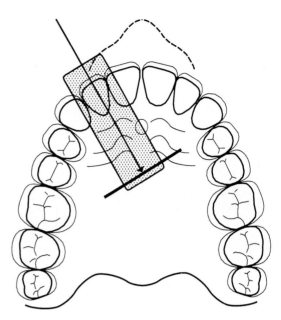

This diagram shows the lateral incisor centered and the film placed well into the oral cavity.

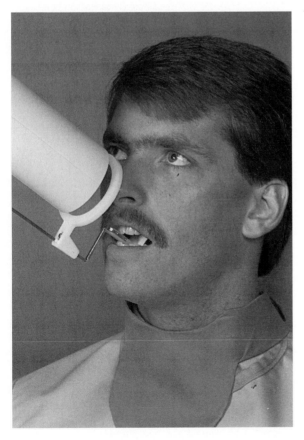

Final positioning of film and instrument. Note that the instrument contacts the tooth of interest and that the opposing teeth also contact the biteblock.

PARALLELING TECHNIQUE

Maxillary Cuspid Region

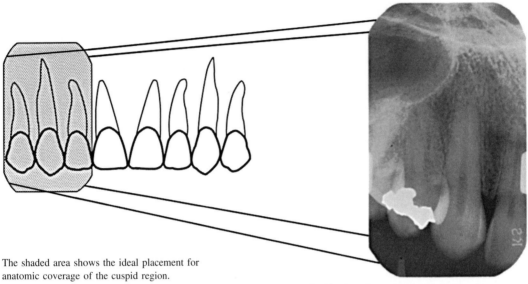

The shaded area shows the ideal placement for anatomic coverage of the cuspid region.

In this view the cuspid is centered on the biteblock. Note that the lingual cusp of the first premolar is superimposed on the distal surface of the cuspid. This superimposition is almost unavoidable because of the maxillary arch curvature, but it should be minimized as much as possible by trying to open the distal contact more than the mesial. This contact area must be "opened" on the next view—the premolar region—seen on the following pages.

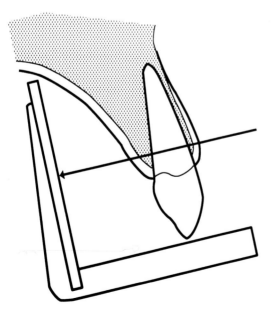

This diagram and the one on the facing page show the positioning of the biteblock near the center of the palate. The central ray is directed perpendicular to the film plane.

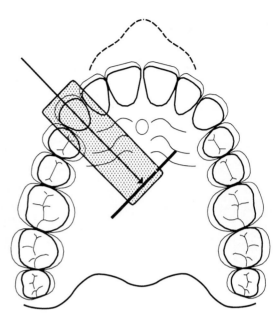

This diagram shows the cuspid centered, and the biteblock placed well into the oral cavity.

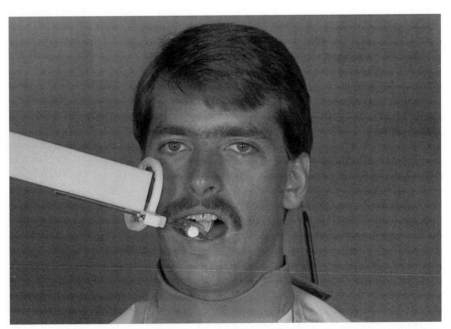

Final positioning of film and instrument. Note that here a rectangular "cylinder" is shown instead of a round one. It is important to rotate the rectangle so that the long dimension is aligned with the film.

PARALLELING TECHNIQUE

Maxillary Premolar Region

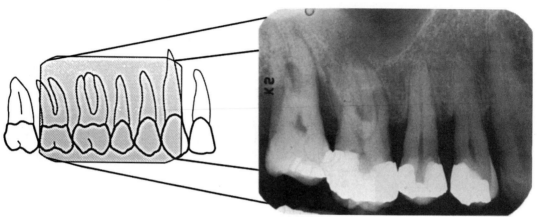

The shaded areas show the ideal placement for anatomic coverage of the premolar and first molar region. Note here that the distal half of the cuspid is visible without overlap, as seen in the typical cuspid view. Size no. 2 film is used in a horizontal orientation.

In this view the contact between the second premolar and first molar is centered on the film.

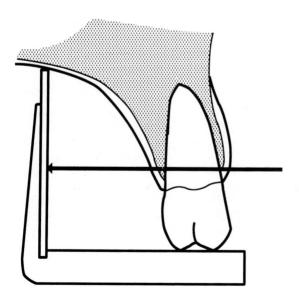

This diagram and the one on the facing page show the positioning of the film near the center of the palate. The central ray is directed perpendicular to the film plane.

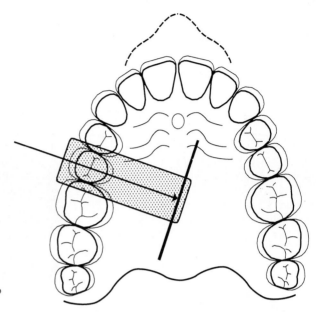

This diagram shows the second bicuspid being centered on the biteblock. The contact between the first molar and the second premolar may also be the centering point.

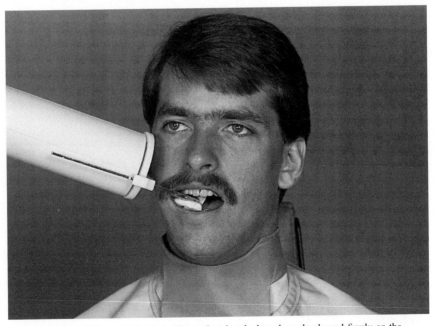

Final positioning of film and biteblock. The patient is asked to close slowly and firmly on the biteblock. Note also that a cotton roll has been placed next to the biteblock on the side opposite the one contacted by the teeth of interest; this technique is used to balance the occlusion. In this example the cuspid would have rocked on the biteblock and would probably have rotated into a less than ideal position. A cotton roll can be placed on the opposite side or surface of any of the films used. The patient is asked to close slowly and firmly onto the biteblock.

PARALLELING TECHNIQUE

Maxillary Molar Region

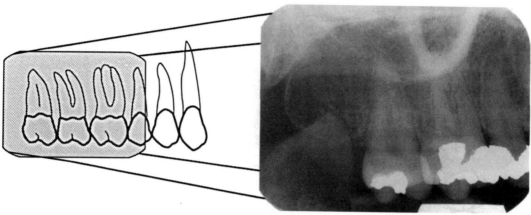

The shaded area shows the ideal placement for anatomic coverage of the molar region. It is important to include *all of the third molar region* in this view.

In this view the second molar is centered on the film. This technique usually ensures complete coverage of the third molar region whether the tooth is present or not.

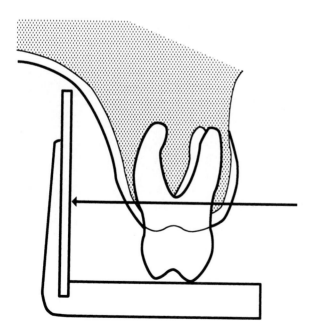

This diagram and the one on the facing page show the positioning of the film near the center of the oral cavity. The central ray is directed perpendicular to the film plane.

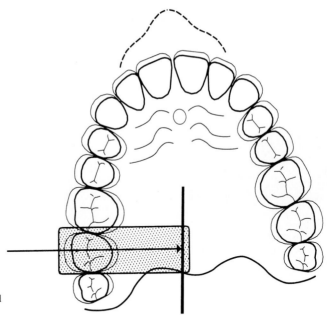

This view shows the second molar centered on the biteblock and on the film.

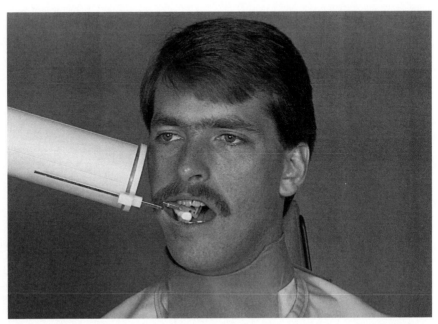

Final positioning of film and biteblock. The patient is asked to close slowly and firmly on the biteblock. Here, too, a cotton roll has been placed on the opposite side of the biteblock for patient comfort and to balance the occlusion. Compare the cylinder position here to that of the maxillary premolar view shown on the previous pages. Note that the cylinder has been placed only slightly more posteriorly for this region.

PARALLELING TECHNIQUE

Mandibular Central Incisor Region

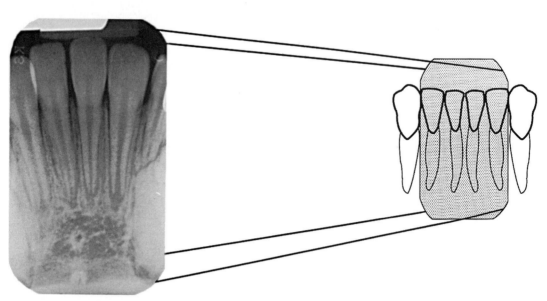

In this view the mandibular incisors are centered approximately on the biteblock. The contact point between the two central incisors would ideally be centered on the biteblock; nevertheless, in this case it is only a minor positioning error, and a retake is not warranted because all of the periapical anatomy of the four incisors is visible.

The shaded area shows the ideal placement for anatomic coverage of the mandibular incisors. Because of their smaller size, all four mandibular incisors can be imaged on a size no. 1 film in a vertical orientation.

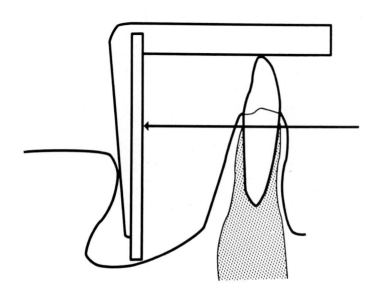

This diagram and the one on the facing page show the film centered on the teeth of interest and contacting the floor of the mouth. The tongue has been slightly displaced by the operator with the film to ensure that the film reaches the floor of the mouth. The central ray is directed perpendicular to the film plane.

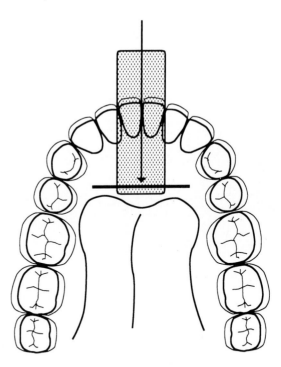

The film is placed as far into the oral cavity as the patient's anatomy will allow. Except in a patient with unusually wide arches, correct positioning rarely results in the films touching or even being close to the lingual surfaces of the teeth.

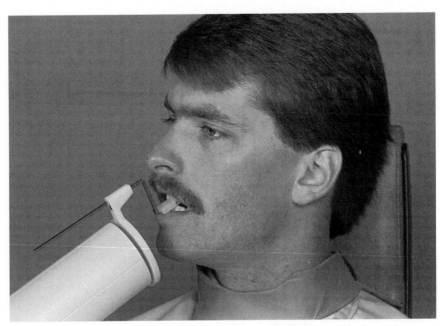

Final positioning of the film and biteblock. Note the negative angulation of the tubehead. The cylinder still parallels the metallic indicating rod, as in the maxillary views.

PARALLELING TECHNIQUE

Mandibular Cuspid Region

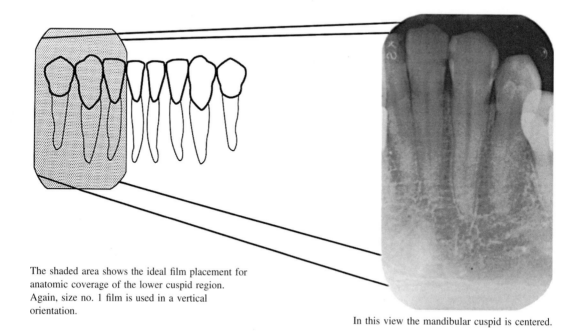

The shaded area shows the ideal film placement for anatomic coverage of the lower cuspid region. Again, size no. 1 film is used in a vertical orientation.

In this view the mandibular cuspid is centered.

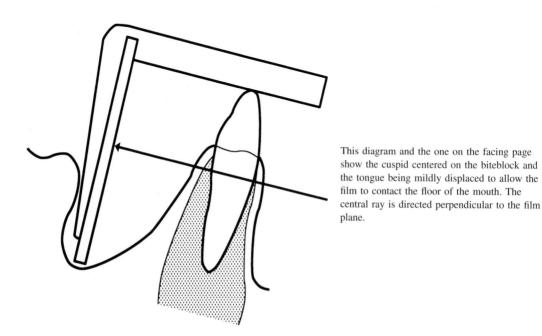

This diagram and the one on the facing page show the cuspid centered on the biteblock and the tongue being mildly displaced to allow the film to contact the floor of the mouth. The central ray is directed perpendicular to the film plane.

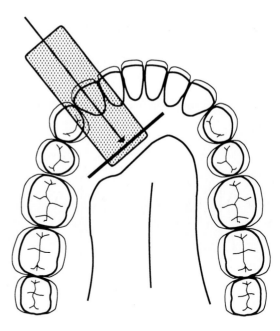

The film is again placed as far into the oral cavity as the patient's anatomy will allow.

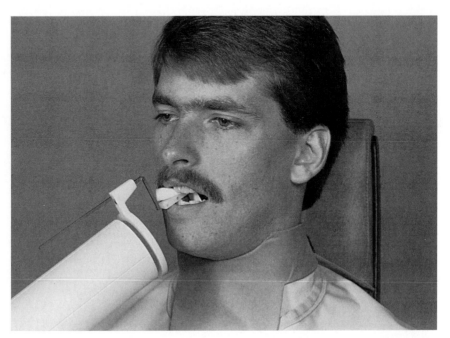

Final positioning of film and biteblock. A cotton roll was used here to prevent rocking of the cuspid cusp tip and displacement of the film. The patient is asked to close slowly and firmly on the biteblock.

PARALLELING TECHNIQUE

Mandibular Premolar Region

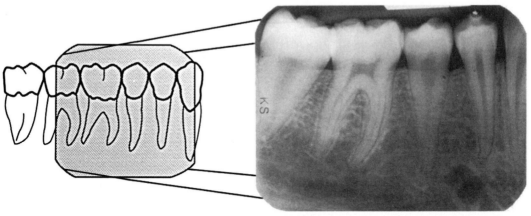

The shaded area shows the ideal film placement for anatomic coverage of the premolar/first molar region. Size no. 2 film is used in a horizontal orientation. As with the maxillary premolar view, it is important to show the distal half of the cuspid in this view.

In this view the contact point between the second premolar and the first molar should be centered.

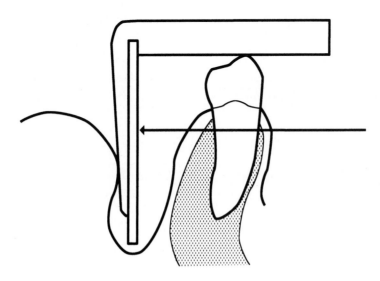

This diagram and the one on the facing page show the biteblock centered on the teeth of interest and the film touching the floor of the mouth.

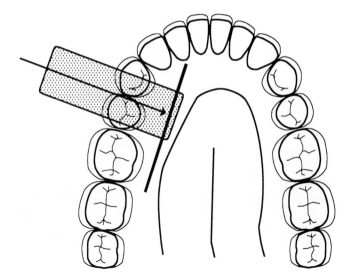

The film is placed as far into the oral cavity as the patient's anatomy will allow.

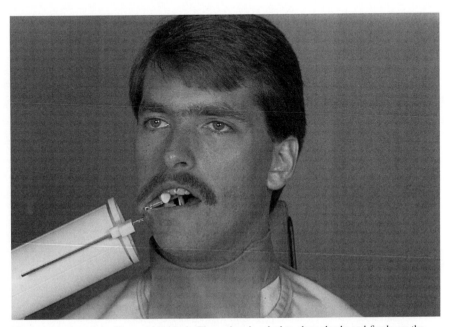

Final positioning of the film and biteblock. The patient is asked to close slowly and firmly on the biteblock.

PARALLELING TECHNIQUE

Mandibular Molar Region

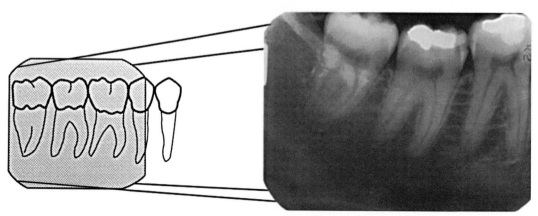

The shaded area shows the ideal film placement for anatomic coverage of the molar region. It is essential to position the film to show all of the *third molar region.*

In this view the second molar has been centered on the film, which allows enough film to be positioned in the third molar region to capture all of that tooth.

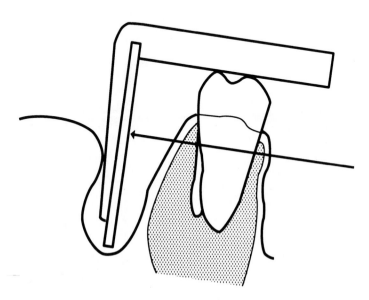

This diagram and the one on the facing page show the biteblock centered on the teeth of interest and the film touching the floor of the mouth. Often more room exists in the floor of the mouth in this region than in the premolar area because of attachments of the mylohyoid muscle.

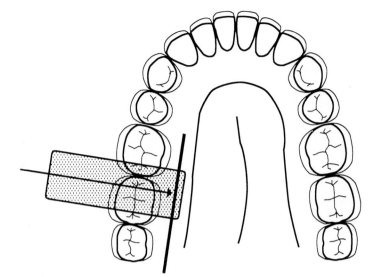

This film is often placed closer to the teeth for the molar view than for premolar and anterior views. The tongue is more difficult to displace in the molar region, and there is sufficient space for the inferior portion of the film to extend into the floor of the mouth.

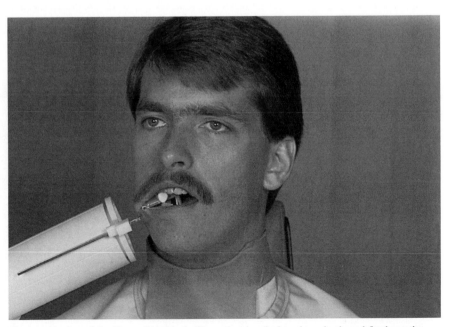

Final positioning of the film and biteblock. The patient is asked to close slowly and firmly on the biteblock.

HELPFUL HINTS FOR INTRAORAL RADIOGRAPHY

Head Position

Position the chair high enough so that you can see the occlusal surfaces of the maxillary teeth when doing maxillary views. Lower the chair when doing mandibular views. Have the patient tilt his or her head slightly backward and open the mouth. Look at the teeth you are going to radiograph. Adjusting the patient's head position is simpler when using indicator rings for alignment. You will not disturb your correct packet placement, and the horizontal and vertical angulation of the beam will be guided by the film-holding device.

Opening Contacts

Before placing anything in the mouth, take a good look at the teeth you are going to radiograph. There are countless ways that the teeth may be rotated or deviated from the normal occlusal pattern. Without knowing what the contact lines between the teeth look like, you cannot be assured of obtaining open contacts on your films. *Never guess!* If you are going to look at the occlusal surfaces of the teeth to try to see the lines made by the contact areas, do not look at them while standing in front of the patient; your view is distorted from that angle. The only way you can obtain a clear view is to stand beside the patient and position yourself so that your eyes are in the same plane that the x-ray beam will be coming from (Fig. 1–34).

If you are looking for mandibular occlusal surfaces, retract the cheek with your finger and look down. If you are looking for the maxillary surfaces, *you cannot see them unless you position your eyes lower than the maxillary occlusal surface and then look straight up.* This means that you are going to have to bend your knees and squat down somewhat as you are looking up.

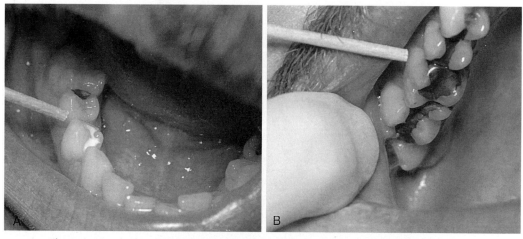

Figure 1–34. *A,* Operator examining contacts of mandibular teeth. *B,* Operator has bent down and is looking up to determine contacts of maxillary teeth. Patient has been asked to tip his head back to assist the operator.

Getting the Film Inside the Mouth

Holding the instrument by the biteblock or the ring, place the film packet inside the mouth. For *maxillary films or bitewings,* tilt the top portion of the film packet toward the center of the mouth, making a "V" shape with the biteblock (Fig. 1–35). This technique keeps you from scraping the film packet across the intraoral tissues. The more you can keep the film packet from scraping across the palate or alveolar ridges, the better your patient will cooperate.

For *mandibular films or bitewings,* you need to lift the tongue out of the way with your index finger so that the lower border of the film packet can slide into place between the tongue and the lingual side of the teeth. Keep the film packet about ¼ inch away from the lingual surface of the teeth. *Do not place the film packet in direct contact with the lingual surface of the teeth.* If you do, you will be inclined to make several technical errors on your film that you will not see until the film is processed. Keeping your finger between the film packet and the alveolar ridge assures that only the soft pad of your finger, not the sharp edge of the film packet, will touch sensitive mucosae as you place the film in the mouth.

Keeping the Film in Place

When you are ready for the patient to bring the teeth together on the biteblock, use this phrase: "*Slowly* close, please." Putting the word "slowly" first, with emphasis, and saying "close" instead of "bite" will give you a chance to keep the film where you placed it and to remove your fingers before the teeth close on them; it will also help the patient to maintain a more relaxed state. Clenching the teeth around the biteblock increases the chances of film bending and of discomfort.

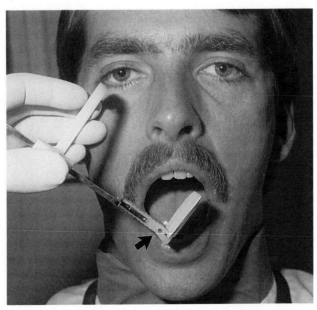

Figure 1–35. The large black arrow points to the "V" shape of the instrument as it is placed into the mouth. Keeping this angle, the operator guides the biteblock up to contact the tooth of interest.

Saying "bite" to a child patient often results in chewing motions from the child, injury to you, and film errors.

Maintaining Patient Cooperation

Place and expose the film as quickly as possible. Remember to turn the unit on and to adjust the exposure settings *before* you place the film in the patient's mouth. Remove the film as soon as it has been exposed. You could even tell the patient to remove the film as soon as the audible signal stops. Taking intraoral radiographs is not a comfortable procedure for many patients. Making the time they have the films in their mouths as short as possible increases their cooperation.

Increasing Success

One of the most common problems that students have with patients is establishing credibility as authority figures. As soon as patients experience the procedure as unpleasant, they begin to question whether it is really necessary. They may also believe, rightly or not, that their discomfort is your fault. To prevent an unpleasant, even argumentative experience,

- **Begin with the easiest films,** probably the maxillary anterior. When these have been exposed successfully, the patient will be more likely to accept that any difficulty with other films is not the fault of an inept radiographer.
- **Be as quick and gentle as possible but speak with authority.** Do not be intimidated. Be sure of what you are doing. If you prepare yourself in advance by learning as much as you can and pay close attention to what you are doing, you have every reason to be confident.

INFECTION CONTROL

No patient should be treated or radiographed without first taking a complete medical history. The medical history has become even more important with the increasing incidence of acquired immunodeficiency syndrome (AIDS) and hepatitis. It should include routine medical questions, a radiation history, and a social history. Certain information elicited from a medical history may alert the radiographer to patients who are "at risk" because of occupation, steroid therapy, certain disease states, a history of an infectious condition, or a lack of cooperation from the patient. Regardless of whether this information is readily available, appropriate infection control procedures are needed for *every* patient to avoid exposure to the operator and cross-infection to other patients.

During a radiographic examination, you will be working directly in the patient's mouth. Immediately after you place the film in his or her mouth, you make the final adjustments of the tubehead and press the exposure button with hands that are now "contaminated." If the x-ray equipment is not properly disinfected or wrapped with barrier material, it is a potential source of cross-contamination.

Sound infection-control procedures, using equipment that has been properly prepared, should be followed.

1. Disinfect and prepare for use all parts of the x-ray unit that will come in contact with the operator's hands during the examination: the control panel, the exposure button, the beam-indicating device (cone), the buttons on the chair, the door handle to the x-ray cubicle, etc. Disinfect flat surfaces on which films are placed. The barrier technique is recommended for any area that has small grooves or hard-to-reach areas such as knobs, buttons, and dials. A piece of plastic wrap works well. Tape may be used to cover the buttons on the chair.
2. Instruments used in the patient's mouth should be sterilized after use with each patient and kept in a closed container for future use.
3. Exposed films should be placed in a paper cup or other disposable container, preferably behind the barrier and *not in the operator's pocket.*
4. The operator should wear gloves and a mask throughout the procedure to protect his or her hands and face.
5. Additional sterilization procedures may be advisable with patients who are identified as being at high risk for transmitting infection.
6. Although there are no vaccinations against tuberculosis, AIDS, or herpes, there is an acceptable vaccine against hepatitis B and D. Dental professionals should give serious thought to the potential consequences of rejecting preventive vaccination because of expense, inconvenience, or fear.

INSTRUCTORS' PRACTICE STRATEGIES FOR STUDENTS

Instrument Assembly Exercise

Students can watch a demonstration of assembly procedures while they assemble their own instruments. Once the assembly is completed, the instructor should have the students disassemble and reassemble the instruments without help. The students should look through the ring to see if the biteblock is centered as a quick check to monitor correct assembly. If video recording equipment is available, the instructor may wish to make a short videotape of the procedure of instrument assembly for the specific positioning devices used at that school. A videotape is helpful because it allows review of the procedure while freeing the instructor for teaching other skills.

Placement Exercise

A videotape of correct placement procedures may be utilized for initial instruction. This videotape will afford each student a good view of the procedure. If a videotape is not available, a demonstration of technique is recommended. Phantoms with tongues are available in many schools. Students may practice instrument placement with the phantoms for specified films and have their film placement checked by the instructor. Alternatively, students may practice placing instruments on each other *without* exposure. Fellow students are very willing to give feedback on the comfort or discomfort of film placement. If this is done, arrangements need to be made in advance to have sterile instruments and gloves available.

Exposing a CMRS or FMX

It is recommended that the first set of radiographs be carefully evaluated but not graded, with as much immediate feedback provided to the student as possible. This procedure will help alleviate some stress for the student trying an unfamiliar procedure. Mistakes can even be encouraged; the opportunity to make errors without being penalized may enable students to learn without frustration. Subsequent surveys should be evaluated as determined by the instructor.

Processing Technique

Expose bitewings and periapicals on a phantom or skull. Save these films to process during the next laboratory session. Films are best kept in a refrigerator if they cannot be processed right away.

Protection Procedures

Describe safety procedures for operators and patients. Using a checksheet of safety procedures, students can watch their lab partners go through the procedure of setting up and making an exposure. When the partner is finished, the observing student can give him or her feedback on any errors, and make corrections. Reverse the procedure for the other partner.

Exposure Factors

Change the exposure factors for each x-ray unit to be utilized in the laboratory. Have one lab partner locate the chart indicating the exposure factors. Instruct him or her to reset the correct factors for each technique listed. Correct any errors.

FINAL WORDS OF ADVICE TO STUDENTS

Remember that radiography is a skill. You will not be proficient immediately— proficiency takes practice. If this were not true, there would be little need to devote so much time to learning and practice. While practicing, you will have access to experts (your instructors) who are available specifically to help you acquire the necessary skills. Take advantage of their expertise. Do not be afraid to ask for guidance and feedback; that is how you learn.

Making mistakes is an important part of the learning process. If you make mistakes during the time you are practicing, someone will be there to give feedback. If you have the opportunity to practice on mannequins, "DEXTERS" (DXTTRS*), or skulls before making films of patients, take advantage of that practice time.

---

*DXTTRS, Dentsply RINN Corporation, Elgin, IL.

Study Questions

1. The embossed dot on the film envelope should always be placed in which direction from the x-ray source?
   A. Away from the source.
   B. Toward the source.
   C. It does not matter.
   D. Away from the source on the mandibular arch and toward the source on the maxillary arch.

2. Which radiographic technique records the most accurate image of crowns, roots, and supporting structures of a selected area?
   A. Bitewing.
   B. Extraoral.
   C. Occlusal.
   D. Periapical.

3. Using the paralleling technique, the central ray makes a right angle (90°) with which structure?
   A. The film.
   B. The long axis of the tooth.
   C. The film and the long axis of the tooth.

4. The *primary* diagnostic use of interproximal (bitewing) radiographs is to
   A. Register the appearance of supporting structures such as bone and soft tissue.
   B. Detect caries and crestal bone levels.
   C. Check for unerupted teeth.
   D. Check crown preparation/placement and residual excess cement.

5. The standard film size used for adult bitewings and posterior periapicals is number
   A. 1
   B. 2
   C. 3
   D. 4
   E. Any of the above size films could be used for bitewings.

6. Correct use of the paralleling technique with film-holding devices offers which of the following technique advantages over the bisecting angle technique without film holders?
   A. Elimination of "cone cuts."
   B. Better film stability.
   C. Less potential for film bending.
   D. Correct angulation between beam and film.
   E. All the above.

7. A no. 1 size film would most likely be used to radiograph which of the following area(s) on an adult patient?
   A. Incisors and canines.
   B. Any area of interest.
   C. Maxillary premolars.
   D. Mandibular premolars if the floor of the mouth is too shallow.

8. The premolar bitewing radiograph should be placed to include which of the following anatomic structures?
   A. All of the maxillary first premolar.
   B. The distal half of the mandibular canine.
   C. The distal half of the maxillary canine.
   D. The mesial half of the maxillary first molar.

9. If you do not have an acceptable barrier between you and the x-ray unit during radiographic procedures, you should
   A. Stand directly behind the x-ray tube with the x-ray beam exiting the tube in the opposite direction from where you are standing.
   B. Stand at a 45 degree angle from the x-ray beam and at least 6 feet away.
   C. Wear a lead apron. Then it will not matter where you stand.
   D. Obtain a monitoring device to keep track of the radiation to which you are being exposed.

10. You have a patient who has read articles describing the hazards of medical/dental radiation and is not sure about letting you take "x-rays" on her. Based on what this chapter describes, what could you explain about your procedures that would be reassuring?
    A. You are using a lead apron and lead thyroid shield.
    B. You are using the long cone paralleling technique.
    C. You take radiographs only when a need is indicated by clinical examination, not based on an arbitrary time schedule.
    D. All of the above.

11. On a premolar periapical, it is critical to obtain which of the following anatomic structures?
    A. Complete view of the premolars and the first molar with an open contact between the premolar and first molar.
    B. Complete view of the premolars and at least one-third of the canine.
    C. Complete view of the premolars plus the first and second molar with an open contact between the two premolars.
    D. Complete view of premolars and the canine. Premolars should be centered on film.

12. Film bending around the apical area is a common problem to watch for and correct on all of the following four views except
    A. Maxillary molars.
    B. Maxillary incisors.
    C. Mandibular premolars.
    D. Bitewings.

13. One of the most common problems associated with correct positioning of mandibular films is
    A. Not having the patient bite hard enough.
    B. Using the wrong size film.
    C. Film bending.
    D. Having the film positioned too close to the lingual side of the teeth.

14. Incorrect horizontal angulation causes
    A. An elongated image.
    B. Overlapped images because the x-ray beam itself is not at a right angle to the film.
    C. Blurred images of the teeth because the x-ray beam is not perpendicular to the long axis of the tooth.
    D. Overlapped images because the lingual aspect of one tooth is superimposed on the facial aspect of the adjacent tooth.

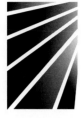

Chapter 2

Film Processing and Quality Assurance

FILM COMPOSITION

Radiographic film is similar to photographic film in many respects. The final image on the film is produced when energy (light or radiation) interacts with the emulsion (chemicals) in the film. To understand film processing, it is necessary to study some basic concepts about the film itself and the chemicals used in processing.

Inside the plastic or paper cover of a film packet, black paper wrapping surrounds the semiflexible plastic film (Fig. 2–1). If you have the opportunity, open a film packet and look at the contents when you read this section.

The plastic film has a green coating of gelatin and chemicals. The film is a series of layers, beginning with a base of thin polyester plastic (Fig. 2–2). The plastic base is transparent but has a blue tint to modulate the bright light transmitted through the film from the view box.

The Emulsion. A coating called the *emulsion* is attached to both sides of the base. The emulsion is a homogeneous mixture of gelatin and grains of silver halide crystals. Silver bromide (AgBr) and silver iodide (AgI) are two types of silver halide used in the emulsion; halides are chemical compounds that change when exposed to light or radiation. These grains of silver halide are suspended in the gelatin similar to the way fruit is suspended in Jell-O. When the silver halide grains are exposed to light or x rays, they store energy from the radiation.

The gelatin is transparent in order to transmit light and porous to allow the processing chemicals to reach the crystals. The gelatin holds the crystals in place until some of the crystals are removed in the fixing process.

Film Speed. How efficiently film responds to radiation determines how much radiation is needed to produce an image. Very efficient film, known as fast or high-speed film, requires less radiation because the film responds more quickly. The two speeds now in use in dentistry are Ultra-speed,* which is also labeled ANSI speed group D, and Ektaspeed Plus,† which is also labeled ANSI speed group E. This information, along with the film size, the number of films in each film packet (one-film packets or two-film packets), and the expiration date, are on the outside of the film box.

The Ektaspeed Plus film is more sensitive (i.e., higher-speed) and may reduce the radiation required for an image by as much as 40 to 50 percent. The higher speed is accomplished primarily by using newer T-grain technology and a different base, which is thinner. This is similar in technology to the Kodak 35-mm photographic film.

LATENT IMAGE FORMATION

Various areas on the film receive more or less radiation, depending on the attenuation differences of the objects irradiated. Another discussion of attenuation

*Ultra-speed, Eastman Kodak, Rochester, NY.
†Ektaspeed Plus, Eastman Kodak, Rochester, NY.

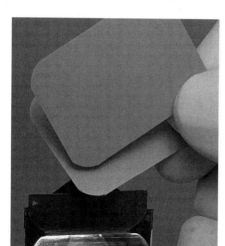

Figure 2–1. Contents of film packet: lead foil, x-ray film, and black paper.

may be found in Chapter 4. In this section, *attenuation* means the way that different tissues stop different numbers of x rays. Thus, exposed films have areas in which silver halide crystals contain various levels of stored energy. The stored energy cannot be seen, but the pattern formed by the energized and nonenergized crystals creates an image within the emulsion. This unseen pattern or image is called the *latent image.*

Pretend you were a white-skinned person wearing a swimming suit made of

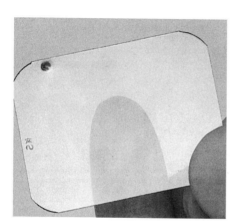

Figure 2–2. Semitransparent, polyester plastic film base. This film has *not* been exposed to radiation. When it was processed, all of the emulsion or chemicals were removed to leave the transparent backing only.

lace and were exposed to the summer sun for 2 hours. The areas where the lace was thick and dense would have stopped the sun's rays. The "see-through" areas would allow the sun to reach your skin. After 2 hours the sunburn probably wouldn't be visible yet, but the image of the lace would be there. This unseen image is the latent image. After about 6 hours, you would probably see the pattern of the lace on your skin. Areas where the lace was see-through would be red (i.e., a maximum amount of sun got through); areas where the lace was thin might be pink (i.e., a medium amount of sun got through); and areas where the lace was thick, or dense, might still be white (i.e., little or no sun got through). This ability of the lace (or the tooth) to absorb different amounts of the radiation based on different densities is called *attenuation.*

The exposed film with its latent image is ready for processing. If the film is never processed, the stored energy will eventually dissipate, and the image will fade. Film should be processed as soon after exposure as possible to avoid any fading. If the film cannot be processed immediately, storage in a refrigerator is recommended until processing can be completed.

CONCEPTS OF FILM PROCESSING— AN OVERVIEW

The chemical reactions of film processing begin with the developer. When the film is placed in the developer, the gelatin softens and swells, and the developer permeates the gelatin to react with *all* of the silver halide crystals. The energized crystals (those that the x rays struck) are easily excited and readily react with the developer chemicals. In simplified terms, the reaction causes the silver halide to separate into bromide (or iodide) and metallic silver, which is black. The black metallic silver precipitates into the gelatin and is deposited on the film. If the x rays have been attenuated (stopped) by a dense object like amalgam, enamel, or bone, then the silver halide crystals are not energized, do not react with the developer, and are washed away. The corresponding area on the film will be white; that is, there will be no reaction in that area of the film.

Recall our analogy of the fruit in the Jell-O. Let's imagine that the emulsion is made up of Jell-O and fruit: the Jell-O is the gelatin and the fruit is the silver halide crystals. All fruit struck by radiation is cooked; all other fruit is not cooked. When the Jell-O is exposed to developer, the developer softens the Jell-O enough to allow the cooked (energized) pieces of fruit to sink to the bottom of the Jell-O (like our black metallic silver, which then adheres to the plastic of the film). The uncooked fruit remains suspended in the Jell-O until the fixing process, when it is removed, or washed away.

FIXATION

In the next step of the film processing, fixer permeates the gelatin, coming in contact with all crystals. The energized crystals that are now "developed" have completed a chemical reaction and are not available for further reaction. The *nonenergized* and *undeveloped* crystals are removed from the emulsion and expelled with the fixer chemicals. The energized and developed crystals are fixed and preserved on the film.

In our Jell-O model, the fixer spreads through the Jell-O, removes all the uncooked fruit, and hardens and shrinks the Jell-O so that the cooked fruit is trapped in place. The uncooked fruit (undeveloped silver halide) floats in the fixer tank and continues to accumulate each time this procedure is followed.

To review, the developer precipitates black metallic silver from *exposed and energized silver halide crystals* into the emulsion, making the dark areas on the film. The fixer removes *unexposed, nonenergized, and undeveloped crystals* from the film, creating the white or clear areas. Therefore, if a film is overexposed or overdeveloped, it will be dark. If a film is underexposed, underdeveloped, or overfixed, it will be light. More information on film and image characteristics appears in Chapter 4.

TECHNICAL ASPECTS OF FILM PROCESSING

The darkroom has tanks of chemicals and water for processing by hand, an automatic processor, or both. Both methods use the same principles and almost identical chemicals. We discuss manual processing first and then describe differences related to automatic processing.

Manual Processing

Film processing refers to the entire sequence of (1) converting the latent (invisible) image to a visible one and (2) preserving the visible image so that it does not disappear later. Because the reactions are chemical, the best results are obtained under optimal conditions.

Developing

Conditions that are of particular importance in developing films are the *temperature of the developer* and the *amount of time* the reaction is allowed to continue. The speed of the developing process depends on the temperature. The higher the temperature, the quicker the development—that is, the shorter the developing time should be. *Optimum developing time and temperature for manual processing is 4½ to 5 minutes at 68°F (20°C).* To ensure proper time and temperature, an accurate thermometer and timer are mandatory (Fig. 2–3).

Consider what would happen if you changed the time but not the temperature. The longer the films were developed, the more the silver halide crystals would precipitate, energized or not. This would cause *all* areas on the film to become darker and less visible. The same thing would happen if you increased the temperature alone. Films developed for 5 minutes at 75°F (24°C) instead of 68°F would be darker. At 68°F, films developed for only 3 minutes would be too light. This may seem like a minor point, but many patients are needlessly overexposed to radiation because of underdevelopment of films. Radiographers may be tempted to increase exposure times when the finished radiograph is too light rather than checking that the developing time and temperature are correct. Using optimum

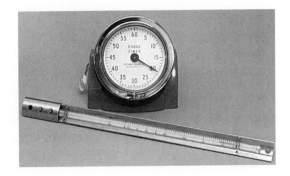

Figure 2–3. Manual timer *(top)* and mercury thermometer. The thermometer sits in the developing tank, for use with either manual or automatic processing techniques.

time and temperature development techniques may significantly reduce x-radiation exposure for patients.

Rinsing

After being developed, the films should be rinsed in clean, circulating water for 30 seconds. Without thorough rinsing of films after development, the fixer will be quickly contaminated with developer, causing problems discussed in the next section.

Fixing Time

The fixing time for manual processing should be at least 10 minutes—that is, twice the usual development time. Fixing for less than 10 minutes or using weak or contaminated fixer will not stop the chemical reaction sufficiently to maintain proper color and clarity for permanent storage; the gray color on the film will eventually turn brown or brownish-yellow, and the transparency of the films will decrease. If films become opaque, they will not transmit light, making them "undiagnostic." Fixer that is not washed off may also cause brown discoloration with age.

If the film has to be viewed right away, it may be read in white light after being developed for 5 minutes and fixed for 3 minutes (i.e., a "wet reading"). The film must then be returned to the fixing bath for 7 minutes more. A word of caution about wet readings: The films are still covered with a coating of fixer, even if they have been rinsed briefly in water. Drops of "water" from these wet films contain residue of fixer and will stain clothing and other films.

Washing and Drying

After the films have been fully fixed, they must be washed and dried. The object of washing is to remove residual processing chemicals and metallic silver from the radiographs. If these chemicals are not removed, the radiograph will discolor with age, impairing its value as a permanent record. Films should be washed in a separate compartment in **clean, running water.** Wash time should be *no less than*

20 minutes, with the circulating water running at a rate sufficient to replace itself every 6 minutes.

After a complete wash, the films are dried. In some offices, films are dried by merely hanging them on a rack in the darkroom above a drip tray. Other offices use an ordinary fan to dry the films. The fan, however, should not blow directly on the films, because lint or dirt may become permanently embedded in the emulsion. Commercial dryers equipped with a fan and a heating element are also available.

Chemicals are available to speed up the drying process. Wetting agents such as Photo-Flo* and Supermix Wetner† are detergents that reduce the surface tension of water, allowing the films to dry faster. Manufacturers' instructions should be followed if these wetting agents are used.

Manual Processing Checklist

In most darkrooms, the developer is in the left tank, the water bath in the center tank, and the fixer in the right tank. *Always* check where everything is before processing. The fixer can be identified, even under a safelight, by its odor and feel. Its acidic properties give it a strong smell similar to vinegar (acetic acid), and it feels slippery.

The steps in manual processing are summarized as follows:

1. **Stir the solutions.** Stirring will equalize the temperature and evenly mix the chemicals. Use different paddles to stir each chemical so that the chemicals will not become contaminated.
2. **Check the solution levels.** If the developer or fixer is low, add the appropriate replenisher. *Do not add water to raise the level.* Solutions that are too low may not completely cover the films attached to the top portion of the film holder, creating artifacts on the films.
3. **Check the temperature of the solutions.** It should be between 65°F (18°C) and 75°F (24°C) if possible; 68–70°F (20–21°C) is optimal. If the temperature is outside this range, regulate the temperature of the running water appropriately, and wait for the chemicals to adjust.
4. **Label the film hanger or rack** with the *patient's name* and the *date of the exposure.* The plastic wrapper from one of the films can be labelled in ballpoint pen and clipped to the film hanger for identification. If more than one film hanger is used, make a separate label for each one.
5. **Turn off the white lights and turn on the safelights.** Until now, the overhead lighting was needed. Check for proper safelighting before opening the film. The way to do this is discussed later.
6. **Remove the exposed film from the packet or cassette.** Clip the film onto the film hanger. *Check to see that the film is clipped tightly* by running your finger along its edge. Residual emulsion on the clips may cause films to become detached and lost in the chemicals. If any of the films are loose, reclip them or put them on another hanger, and check later to see how the problem can be corrected.
7. **Set the timer** according to the temperature of the developer and the

---

*Eastman Kodak Company, Rochester, NY.
†General Electric Company, Milwaukee, WI.

manufacturer's recommendations. *Optimum time/temperature processing is 68°F (20°C) for 4½ or 5 minutes.* If rapid-processing chemicals are used, consult the manufacturer's recommendations. A chart should be posted next to the tanks with correct developing temperatures and appropriate developing times.

8. **Immerse the film in the developer, and start the timer.** Agitate the film hanger to break up residual air bubbles and to allow the developer to completely engulf the films.
9. **When the timer goes off, remove the films and rinse them in running water** in the rinse tank by agitating the film hanger up and down for approximately 15 to 20 seconds.
10. **Immerse the film hanger in the fixer tank** and agitate for approximately 5 seconds. *Set the timer for 10 minutes.* If the films need to be viewed quickly, they can be removed from the fixer after 3 minutes. However, they *must* be returned to the fixer for 7 minutes more.
11. **Wash the films in circulating water for 20 to 30 minutes.** Although the timing of the wash is not as critical as that for developing and fixing, the minimum wash time is 20 minutes. The water must be circulating such that the water in the tank changes every 6 minutes. There is no maximum wash time, but the longer the film is in the water, the softer the emulsion will get. Eventually, the emulsion could be washed off completely: films left in the water overnight are usually blank the next day.
12. **Remove the films from the wash, and place them in a dryer or hang over a drip pan** in a place where they will remain undisturbed until thoroughly dry.
13. **When the films are dry, place them in an appropriately labeled mount.** The mount should have the *patient's name,* the *date* the films were exposed, and the *radiographer's name.*

CHEMICAL COMPOSITION OF SOLUTIONS

Both the developer and the fixer are made up of specific chemicals that serve particular functions. Tables 2–1 and 2–2 are charts of the chemicals and their functions.

TABLE 2–1. DEVELOPER COMPOSITION

FUNCTION	CHEMICAL	CHEMICAL ACTIVITY
Activator	Sodium carbonate	Swells and softens the emulsions so that the reducing agents may work more effectively.
Reducing agents	Metol	Builds up gray tones quickly.
	Hydroquinone	Builds up black tones more slowly than Metol, giving better contrast to the blacks and whites.
Restrainer	Potassium bromide	Keeps the reducing agents from developing unexposed, unenergized silver halide.
Preservative	Sodium sulfite	Prevents rapid oxidation of the other chemicals.
Solvent	Water	Dissolves chemicals.

TABLE 2–2. FIXER COMPOSITION

FUNCTION	CHEMICAL	CHEMICAL ACTIVITY
Acidifier	Acetic or sulfuric acid	Stops development by neutralizing developer; provides required acidity.
Fixing agent	Ammonium thiosulfate	Clears away the unexposed silver halide crystals.
Hardener	Aluminum chloride or sulfide	Shrinks and hardens the emulsion.
Preservative	Sodium sulfite	Maintains chemical balance of the fixer chemicals.
Solvent	Water	Dissolves chemicals.

CARE OF SOLUTIONS

Daily Care/Quality Assurance (QA)

Each day before any patient films are processed, the chemicals should be checked for quality. This will reduce needless patient exposure to radiation because of processing problems. The check can be done using two "checker films" and a homemade stepwedge. A stepwedge is a device with small, graduated increases in the thickness of its material (usually aluminum, if a commercial product). When placed over an x-ray film and exposed, the stepwedge produces a gradient of gray tones on the film from very dark (where the material is thin) to very light (where the material is thick). The thin portion allows many more x rays to pass through it; thus, more film emulsion is exposed. This area of the film will be black. The thick portion attenuates, or stops, x rays; thus, this area of the film will appear lighter. A simple stepwedge using lead foil can be constructed as described later.

Simple Daily QA

1. Process an *unexposed* film. This film should be clear. If not, the cause of the problem should be identified and corrected before proceeding. Problems are usually caused by light "leaks" in the darkroom or by chemical fog owing to outdated or improperly stored film.
2. Expose a checker film using a stepwedge and your usual exposure factors. Process the film. This daily checker film should be compared with a control film. If there is no visible difference, the patient's films can be processed. The control film is made using the same stepwedge and fresh chemicals (see following).

How To Construct a Stepwedge

To make the stepwedge, tape six pieces of lead foil from the inside of the film packets to the end of a tongue blade. The first two pieces should be approximately 1 inch long, the second two approximately ¾ inch long, and the third two approximately ½ inch long. Tape these foil pieces in three steps, with one step having six layers, the second having four layers, and the third having two layers of lead. Cut the excess foil from the sides and tape the foil layers to the tongue blade (Fig. 2–4).

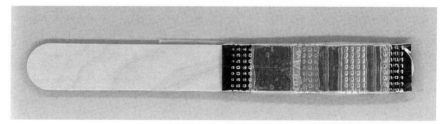

Figure 2–4. Tongue depressor or blade, with foil adapted and taped.

How To Make a Control Film

A control film must be made in fresh solutions. Place a film on a flat surface, such as the arm of the dental chair, with the dot up. Place the stepwedge on top of the film, and set the beam-indicating device over the film (Fig. 2–5). Expose the film, using the setting for a molar bitewing. Process the film in fresh solutions as usual. The control film should be dated and taped to a view box for reference until the solutions are changed again and a new control film is made. Checker films made on a daily basis are compared with this control film.

Checker Film. A checker film should be exposed at the beginning of every day and compared with the control film. It is not acceptable for the checker film to be visibly different from the control film. If there is a visible difference, patient films should not be processed until the source of the problem is identified and corrected. Poor quality checker films may indicate contaminated solutions, weak solutions, or mechanical problems in the equipment (Fig. 2–6).

Preparation and Mixing

Developer and fixer solutions can be prepared from powders or concentrated liquids that are mixed with water, or they may come premixed. Regardless of the

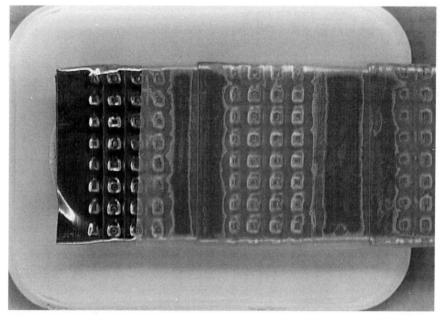

Figure 2–5. Stepwedge placed over x-ray film.

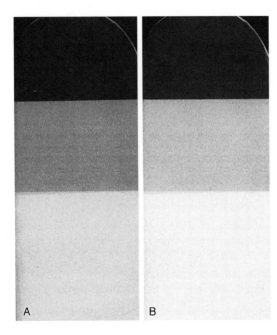

Figure 2–6. A, Image of step-wedge properly exposed in fresh solutions. *B*, Weak or depleted developer solution has produced this lighter stepwedge image.

type used, manufacturer's instructions should be followed. Each set of chemicals has instructions enclosed in the package or printed on the bottles. If the same chemicals are used consistently, it is wise to post a copy of the mixing instructions near the tanks or processor for reference.

Replenishing Chemicals

As the chemicals are used, they lose their effectiveness. They weaken with use, exposure to air, or contamination with water or another processing chemical. Poor quality films may result from inadequate care of the chemicals. To guarantee the highest quality films, the chemicals should be replenished as they are used:

Developer. It is recommended that 6 ounces of developer be added to a 1-gallon tank each morning, whether the tank has been used or not. If the tank solution is at its maximum volume, *6 ounces* of developer should be removed before adding the replenisher. After the replenisher is added, the developer must be stirred to avoid uneven developing. Developer replenisher may be normally prepared developer solution or a special mixture, as specified by the manufacturer. Manufacturer's instructions on preparing replenisher should be followed.

Fixer. Replenishment of the fixer is not as critical as replenishment of the developer. However, even though it may not be necessary to replenish the fixer daily, it may be beneficial to maintain the same schedule for both solutions to ensure that replenishment of the fixer is not forgotten. If the tank solution is at its maximum volume, *3 ounces* of fixer should be removed before replacing with 3 ounces of replenisher. The fixer should also be stirred upon replenishing. Manufacturer's instructions on preparing replenisher should be followed. Keeping the fixer at proper strength will assure adequate clearing and hardening of the emulsion. Replenishment of the chemicals should be incorporated into the daily maintenance routine.

Changing Chemical Solutions

Even though replenishment will prolong the life of the chemicals, this procedure should not be repeated indefinitely. **Changing the chemicals completely is necessary on a regular basis.**

Some people change the processing chemicals according to a time schedule. This is acceptable if the time period does not go beyond the life of the chemicals, which is affected by the number of films processed, the amount of exposure to air, the replenishment schedule, and dilution with water or other chemicals. These factors can vary from office to office, causing some chemicals to be thrown away before necessary and others to be used after they are exhausted. The greatest hazard lies in the temptation to increase the exposure time when films are consistently light without checking the quality of processing solutions. As a result, patients receive unnecessary radiation.

An alternative to changing the solutions according to a time schedule is to rely on the appearance of the checker film. This method was described earlier under "Daily Care." If there is a visible difference in the density on the checker film, the solutions should be changed. If it seems that the solutions are changed quite frequently with this process, they may have been replenished inadequately—that is, either too infrequently or in insufficient amounts. The temperature of the solutions may have damaged the chemicals, or the chemicals may have been exposed to air. These problems are usually easily identified and corrected.

THE DARKROOM

Standard Requirements

The darkroom should be clean, efficient, and well-equipped. Spots, streaks, film fog, and other artifacts on the processed radiograph can often be traced to poor darkroom conditions and uncleanliness. Although it is a tempting place to store film, the darkroom is not recommended for this purpose because of potential reactions between chemical fumes and the film emulsion, resulting in chemical film fog (an overall graying of the film).

There should be adequate space for working, particularly at the counter where films are unwrapped and loaded onto a film rack. The temperature of the room should never exceed 90°F (32°C); temperatures higher than this would be harmful to both the chemicals and the film. A temperature of 70–80°F (21–27°C) at 70 percent humidity is recommended. Inadequate humidity can cause film artifacts, as we will discuss later.

Adequate equipment should include the following:

1. A "light-tight" room with a revolving or locking door or maze and with no cracks around doors, corners, or cabinets that would allow light leaks.
2. Hot and cold running water, with mixing valves to adjust the temperature.
3. Processing tanks and film hangers or racks.
4. A source of white light and *proper* safelights at the appropriate distance from the work surface (at least 4 feet).
5. A timer that is accurate *in minutes and seconds.*
6. An accurate nonmercury thermometer that is easy to read and is kept

submerged in the developer. The mercury in a thermometer will permanently damage the tanks if it comes into contact with the metal lining the tanks.

7. Adequate storage space for chemicals, film hangers, and cassettes.
8. A film-drying rack and a film dryer.

An automatic processor and film duplicator are recommended as standard equipment. If they are not available, space for their future placement should be allowed.

Lighting

The darkroom should be totally dark when all the lights are off. White light may "leak" into the room through any opening such as the door, joints in walls, partitions, keyholes, and air vents. Damaged safelights may also be a source of light leaks. If the darkroom door is not a revolving type, it should have a lock to eliminate accidental opening. Some darkroom entryways employ a maze of walls rather than a door. These are usually "lightproof."

Some types of fluorescent lights have a short afterglow that could fog the first few films opened after the room light has been turned off. These should be replaced. Although extraneous light should be eliminated, the room should contain a source of white light (regular room lighting) and a safelight, each with its own switch. It is also desirable to have an illuminator (view box) in the darkroom.

Safelights are devices that provide enough illumination in the darkroom to work by and to process films without danger of fogging the film. X-ray film is sensitive to both radiation and visible light (white light); it is most sensitive to blue and green light and least sensitive to yellow and red light. Consequently, safelights usually contain regular light bulbs with red, yellow, or brown filters covering the bulb. These remove or filter out the light to which the film is most sensitive, the light in the blue-to-green range.

Commercially available darkroom filters include the Kodak Morlite* (ML-2), which is a light orange filter, closer to green than to red in the light spectrum; it transmits the most light. As a result, it is easier to work using this filter because of the greater visibility. However, this filter cannot be used with extraoral films, because they are sensitive to light nearer the green part of the light spectrum and would be fogged.

The Kodak GBX* is a red filter that, unlike the Kodak Morlite, can be used in darkrooms in which both intraoral and extraoral films are processed. It filters out light nearer the green-to-blue spectrum, thus protecting sensitive extraoral films.

All film is somewhat sensitive to any light. In order to avoid light fogging, bulb wattage and distance to the work surface have to be regulated. If the safelighting is direct (the light shining down upon the work surface), the bulb should be no brighter than 15 watts. If the safelighting is indirect (the light shining up toward the ceiling and then reflecting down), the bulb should be no brighter than 25 watts. The distance from the light to the workbench should be at least 4 feet, regardless of whether direct or indirect illumination is used.

Quality assurance in checking the darkroom for light leaks and proper safelights is simple. To check for light leaks around the doors, lights, walls, windows, vents, etc., simply go into the darkroom and turn off *all* the lights. Wait 2 or 3 minutes

*Eastman Kodak, Rochester, NY.

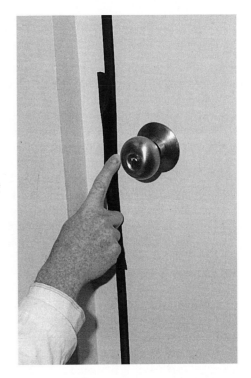

Figure 2–7. Tape being applied to area of "light leak."

for your eyes to adjust to the darkness. Then look around the room carefully. If you see light coming from anywhere, you have a light leak that should be corrected (Fig. 2–7).

Coin Test

The "coin test" can be used to check the safelights. With the safelights on and the white light off, unwrap a piece of film. Lay it on the counter and place a coin in the center. Wait between 3 and 5 minutes (approximately the time it would take you to unwrap a CMRS (FMX), load it onto a rack, and place it in the developer). Process the film as usual. If the image of the coin is visible, light is coming from somewhere to fog (expose) the film. Safelight bulbs should be checked for correct wattage, the lights should be measured for correct distance, and the filters should be checked for cracks.

AUTOMATIC FILM PROCESSING

Manual processing for intraoral films is gradually being replaced by the automatic processor for a number of reasons:

1. Automatic processors can shorten the processing time to as little as a total of 4 to 5 minutes.
2. The automatic processing cycle produces consistently good end results if the equipment and chemicals are properly maintained. In addition, there is less opportunity for operator error.

3. Automatic processors usually require less space than manual equipment, and some have daylight loading capability that does not require a darkroom.

An automatic processor is usually constructed of a series of rollers that transport the films through various compartments (developer, fixer, rinse water) and a blower to dry the films (Fig. 2–8).

The processor contains a heating element that maintains a constant temperature in the developer. The rollers are set to rotate at a speed according to the temperature of the developer in order to produce optimal films. Although this mechanisms can also be thought of as time/temperature developing, the temperatures of the developer in automatic processors range from 85°F to 105°F (29°C to 40°C), significantly reducing the developing time and the overall processing procedure.

While moving the film through the processor, the rollers provide a massaging action that contributes to the speed and uniformity of processing. In addition to these transport rollers, special squeegee rollers remove processing solutions from the film surfaces, reducing the amount of "solution carryover" from one tank to the next. This process prolongs the life of the fixer and removes most of the wash water from the film emulsion before the film enters the drying section. Warm, dry air is blown onto the film before it exits the processor at the receiving tray.

Because the total time is reduced in automatic processing, the chemical concentration and temperature of the solutions must be increased. The automatic processor commonly used in dentistry maintains temperatures of approximately 83–85°F (28–29°C) for a 4½- to 5-minute cycle. For larger, 90-second processing machines, the developing temperature is about 95–101°F (35–38°C).

To prevent the emulsion from softening and sticking to the rollers, a special hardening chemical, glutaraldehyde, is added to the developer. Sulfate compounds are also added to the developer to minimize the swelling of the emulsion. If the emulsion has absorbed too much developer, the films will get stuck in the rollers.

Maintenance of Automatic Processors

A rigid schedule for replenishment is far more critical with automatic processors. For example, weak fixer will not shrink the emulsion enough to keep the film moving through the rollers. Films may stick in the fixer or dryer rack, impeding the path of following films.

Automatic processors also demand routine preventive maintenance. Experience has shown that the two greatest causes of automatic processor breakdown are (1) failure to keep the rollers clean and (2) inadequate replenishing. A schedule should

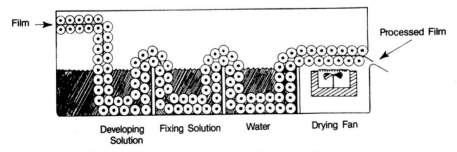

Film →   Processed Film

Developing   Fixing Solution   Water   Drying Fan
Solution

Figure 2–8. Schematic drawing of typical automatic film processor.

be established for daily clearer films and replenishment as well as for monthly cleaning and solution changes. Guidelines appropriate to maintenance of all automatic processors follow:

Replenishment. Solutions should be replenished at the beginning of each day, regardless of amount of use, and a regular basis according to the number of films processed. After four CMRS, or panoramic, films, 4 to 6 ounces of processing chemicals should be added. Failure to add this amount will result in exhausted developer and fixer and, consequently, undiagnostic radiographs.

Cleaning the Rollers. The rollers should be cleaned with warm running water *weekly.* The rollers should be soaked for approximately 10 to 15 minutes before being placed back in the processor. Two extraoral-size "cleaning" films should be run through the processor before patient films are processed.

Changing Solutions. The solutions should be changed *every 2 to 6 weeks,* depending on the rate of use and the frequency of replenishment. It is wise to empty only one compartment at a time, beginning with the fixer. Cleaning solutions recommended by the manufacturer should be used. If there are no recommendations, or if those solutions are not available, the following cleaning solutions can be used: (1) special developer cleaner for the developing racks and compartment; (2) warm running water for the fixer rollers and compartment; and (3) mild household bleach solutions for the wash compartment. All racks should be rinsed thoroughly with warm running water before they are put back in the processor. The stopper or plug should be removed from one compartment at a time. Each compartment should be totally cleaned and rinsed and *the stopper replaced* before proceeding. This will prevent backflow of chemicals into the wrong compartment. After thorough cleaning, each compartment should be filled with clear water and the processor run for approximately 5 to 10 minutes. After the water is drained, the fixer should be replaced first, followed by the developer. If the developer splashes accidentally into the fixer, the contamination is not as damaging as when the reverse occurs.

Monthly Cleaning. Monthly cleaning includes cleaning the rollers, as described in the section on changing solutions. This is also the time to check the unit (particularly the dryer) for dust and to lubricate moving parts.

Helpful Hints

The most important factor in maintaining the processor is regular preventive maintenance. The following suggestions are to help prevent problems commonly associated with automatic processors:

1. Keep the cover open slightly, particularly over the motor, when the processor is *not in use.* Accumulated fumes will fog films if not vented, and the moisture around the motor will cause premature rusting and breakdown. Be sure to replace the cover tightly before processing films.
2. Lubricate the moving parts as indicated in the owner's manual.
3. Check the temperature of the solutions regularly. A few degrees' difference in the developer temperature will change the density of the films.
4. Check each day to see that the rollers are locked in proper position to prevent the loss of films.
5. *Replenish the chemicals* as described previously.

6. Feed the films slowly into the machine and keep them straight. If they turn sideways even slightly, they may merge and stick together.
7. Count 10 to 15 seconds after feeding each film into the processor before inserting another film.
8. Alternate slots or sides when possible.
9. Check to be sure that the black paper has been removed and double-pack films have been separated, and place only the films into the processor.
10. Do *not* put wet films into the processor, as they will contaminate the rollers.

TROUBLESHOOTING: DIAGNOSING PROCESSING ERRORS

Processed films may not be as good as expected. Table 2–3 lists different problems, possible causes, and appropriate corrections. *Most* of these conditions pertain to both manual and automatic processing. Exposure errors and radiographic examples of errors that may cause similar appearances are discussed in Chapter 5.

MOUNTING FILMS

Instructions on film mounting will be discussed in Chapter 11.

Preparing the Mount

Processed films are normally placed in a film holder, either cardboard or plastic, that arranges the films in an anatomically oriented pattern and protects them from scratches and careless handling. Mounting films routinely and correctly reduces the potential for incorrect interpretation, such as confusing the right side with the left.

Looking at a *set* of films is also more efficient than viewing one at a time. Although each film is viewed individually, an overview of the complete survey gives the operator the opportunity to look for symmetry and to compare sides for bone pattern, eruption sequences, size and shape of teeth, etc. (Fig. 2–9).

The mount should be opaque to eliminate extraneous light from around the films. Eliminating extraneous light enables the eye to detect the subtle differences in density that may indicate the presence or absence of pathology. The film mount (Fig. 2–10A) should contain the right number and size frames to hold the prepared films. Empty frames should be blocked out with opaque material such as film blanks (Fig. 2–10B).

The film mount should be labeled *before* use. If films become separated from the patient's chart, they cannot be identified if they are not labeled. The information on the mount should include three things:

1. *The patient's full name,* not just the last name and initial.
2. *The date the films were exposed.* Even if the films are processed on a different date, the exposure date should be the one recorded on the mount. This is a radiographic record of the patient's intraoral condition on the date of the exposure, not on the processing date.

TABLE 2-3. TROUBLESHOOTING FOR PROCESSING ERRORS

CONDITION	POSSIBLE CAUSES	WHAT TO DO
1. Light films (low density or contrast)	A. Underdevelopment	
	1. Temperature too low	Check temperature.
	2. Time too short	Check time (if possible).
	3. Inaccurate thermometer or timer	Check timer and thermometer.
	B. Exhausted developer	Do checker film.*
	C. Diluted developer	Do checker film.
2. Dark films (high density)	A. Overdevelopment	
	1. Temperature too high	Check temperature.
	2. Time too long	Check time.
	3. Inaccurate thermometer or timer	Check thermometer and timer.
	B. Light leak in darkroom or processor	Check inside darkroom.* Do coin test.
	C. Exposure of films to white light.	Turn overhead lights off.
3. Grayish films (film fog)	A. Light leaks	Check inside darkroom for leaks.* Do coin test.
	B. Improper or defective safelights	Check safelights* for correct wattage or light leaks due to cracks.
	C. Exposure of films to white light before complete fixing	
	D. Exposure of films to unwanted radiation	Check storage area of films and check for films left in x-ray cubicle while exposing.
	E. Chemical fog Overdevelopment (time)	Check temperature (it may have increased and changed development time).
	F. Outdated film	
4. Yellow or brown films	A. Exhausted developer	Do checker film.*
	B. Exhausted fixer	Do checker film.*
	C. Incomplete fixing	Check fixing time.
	D. Insufficient washing	Rewash.
5. Streaks	A. Careless rinsing before fixing	
	B. Exhausted chemicals	Do checker film.*
	C. Contaminated developer or wash water	Do checker film.
	D. Contaminated rollers	Run cleaning film through processor; clean rollers if necessary.
6. Greenish films	A. Contaminated or exhausted fixer	Replenish or change fixer.
	B. Insufficient washing	Rewash.
	C. Films stuck together (uneven developing)	Replace in fixer and continue processing.
7. Black or white lines	A. Film bending	Look for bend. Curve but do not crease film if possible.
	B. Rough film handling	
8. Lightening or tree-like marks (static electricity)	A. Excessively dry air (most commonly seen on extraoral films)	Humidify darkroom. Use Static Guard on clothing/hair.
9. Spots	A. Water droplets on film	Check counter for cleanliness.
	B. Premature contact with developer (black spots)	Check counter for cleanliness.
	C. Premature contact with fixer (white spots)	Check counter for cleanliness.

*See section on quality assurance for specific checks and tests.

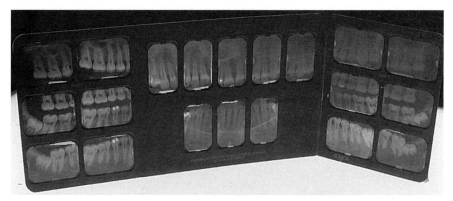

Figure 2–9. Complete set of periapical and bitewing radiographs.

3. *The name of the radiographer.* This is the person who may be able to furnish information should future questions arise. Recording the name also gives a quality of "ownership" for a skill performed and a means of quality assurance for technique. The radiographer may be a little more particular with technique if his or her name is attached for others to see. If the operator is consistently making the same error, remediation may be in order. Thus, the error can be identified and the operator can be given instructions for correction.

DUPLICATING FILMS

For many reasons a practitioner may desire a copy or duplicate set of radiographs. Preauthorization for treatment, population mobility, and protection from liability may dictate the need for more than one copy of a radiographic survey.

Intraoral films are available in double-film packets—that is, two pieces of film in one packet. They are exposed in the normal manner, and the films are separated prior to processing. This way two identical sets of films are obtained with no extra radiation exposure for the patient.

An alternative method is to copy the radiographs using duplicating film and a film duplicator as shown in Figure 2–11. Duplicating film has emulsion on one side only and is sensitive to light, particularly ultraviolet light. The reaction of the

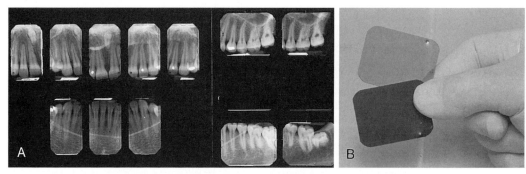

Figure 2–10. *A,* Opaque x-ray mount, with appropriate areas filled with black films to mask extraneous light. *B,* The film blank, which appears black in this figure, is used for this purpose.

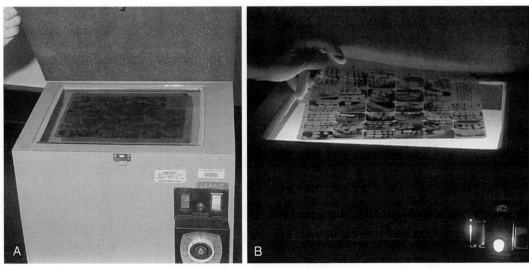

Figure 2–11. Two types of film duplicator.

emulsion is the opposite of that of radiographic film. When exposed to radiation or light, x-ray film becomes dark. Duplicating film, on the other hand, becomes lighter with increasing exposure to light.

Duplication is performed in the darkroom under safelights. Radiographs are placed on a duplicator, and the duplicating film is placed carefully on top with the emulsion side (which is normally gray or lavender) against the radiographs. If available, film organizers, which look similar to film mounts but are especially designed for duplicating, should be used to organize the films (Fig. 2–12). The organizers are helpful because they blacken the areas around each film, eliminating extraneous light transmission.

In the duplicator there is a source of light (usually ultraviolet). The light passes through the original radiograph and strikes the duplicating film. Light areas of the radiograph allow increased light transmission to the duplicating film. The longer the duplicating film is exposed to light, the lighter the duplicate films will become. This is the opposite of x-ray films, which become darker when exposed to light.

This process is also helpful in producing acceptable radiographic copies (Fig. 2–13A) of films that are underexposed and too light or overexposed and too dark to interpret (Fig. 2–13B). However, making darker duplicates of overly light radiographs is not as successful.

The duplicating film is then processed normally. If the duplicates are not as good as the original films, the process can be repeated without additional radiation exposure to the patient.

Helpful Hint

It is very important to obtain good contact between the duplicating film and the radiographs to prevent blurring and fuzziness of the image. Regular film mounts should not be used as film organizers because they hold the radiograph away from the duplicating film slightly, preventing good contact. They also "cut off" the edges of the films, leaving an incomplete view. The radiograph should be placed

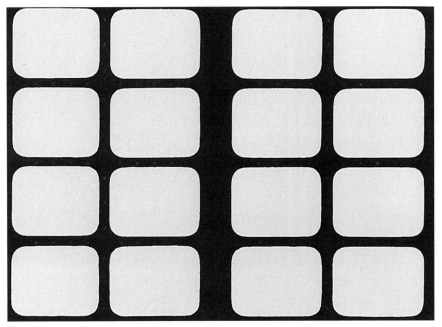

Figure 2–12. X-ray "organizer" on which to place films for duplication. Films to be duplicated are centered in the clear area, and an edge of the film is taped lightly to hold them in place when the duplicating film is placed over them.

on the duplicator with the dot downward in order to make good contact with the duplicating film. Care should be taken to ensure that the original radiographs are arranged in the correct position. No raised dot exists on the duplicating film to identify films that may have been mounted incorrectly. The duplicate film should be labeled *immediately* with the patient's name, the date the originals were made, and which side is right or left.

STUDENT PRACTICE AND INSTRUCTOR RECOMMENDATIONS

To the instructor: Following are laboratory exercises that students can perform with or without instructor supervision. Sets of practice films can be prepared by

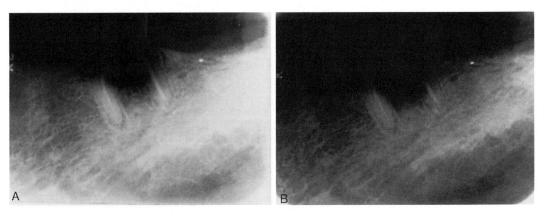

Figure 2–13. *A,* This film was duplicated from the dark film seen in *B.* More detail is seen in *A,* especially around the root tips.

the instructor in advance for the students to use. The exercise may be self-paced and self- or instructor-evaluated. Group practice with continuous instructor feedback may also be used.

Using one set, students are given feedback for learning purposes. Using a second set, students are checked for competency before progressing to another task. Several sets of the same films may be made using duplicating film, offering each student the same learning experience.

Processing

1. Students should process films exposed on a phantom. If possible, process half of the films manually and half of the films with an automatic processor. Have the students prepare a list of the advantages and disadvantages of each method.
2. Using a set of preprocessed films with specific processing errors, have the students identify the errors on each film. Discuss the films with the students or have them check the answers against a master key.

A second set may be used for checking competency. Additional sets or exercises may be given until the student has mastered the task.

Mounting

Provide a set of films and a mount for the students to practice mounting the films. After they complete the practice set, a different set may be used to check for competency.

Study Questions

1. The latent image on a radiograph is
   A. An unseen image produced by silver halide crystals that have been exposed to radiation and contain various levels of stored energy, making a pattern.
   B. The image seen on the film after removal of the unexposed silver halide crystals in the developing solution.
   C. The image seen on the film after removal of the exposed silver halide crystals in the developing solution.
   D. The image seen on the film after the film has been in the fixer at least 3 minutes.
2. Film speed is determined by
   A. The size of the film packet.
   B. The amount of radiation emitted from the x-ray machine.
   C. The exposure time.
   D. The size of the silver halide crystals.

3. During the chemical processing procedure, the fixer
   A. Removes the metallic silver deposited during the developing process.
   B. Removes the unexposed silver halide crystals, leaving white (or clear) spots where those crystals used to be.
   C. Precipitates the exposed (energized) crystals onto the base of the film, forming the black areas.
   D. Softens the emulsion in order to "set" energized crystals and remove nonenergized crystals.

4. The optimum developing time and temperature for manual processing is
   A. 68°F (20°C) for 4½ to 5 minutes.
   B. 68°F (20°C) for 10 minutes.
   C. 85°F (29°C) for 90 seconds.
   D. 95° to 105°F (35°C to 40°C) for 20 to 30 seconds.

5. A stepwedge (or x-ray checker) may be used to
   A. Check the quality of the processing chemicals.
   B. Check the darkroom for light leaks.
   C. Determine processing times when chemical temperatures vary.
   D. Determine the speed of the film.

6. The emulsion is softened, and exposed silver halide crystals precipitate from within the gelatin onto the film base during the
   A. Latent period.
   B. Developing cycle.
   C. Fixing cycle.
   D. Washing cycle.

7. Which of the following is not a characteristic of an ideal film mount?
   A. Translucency in order to transmit more light to enhance viewing.
   B. The right number and size of frames for the films taken.
   C. Providing a place for the operator's name, patient's name, and exposure date.
   D. Fitting into the patient's chart.

8. After you have processed a checker film in an automatic processor prior to processing any patient films, you find the checker film to be light. The temperature was appropriate for the developing time. There is no log of how long the chemicals have been used. Which of the following is an appropriate step to take?
   A. Increase the exposure time to darken the films.
   B. Change the chemicals.
   C. Increase the fixing time.
   D. Increase the developing time.

9. After doing a "coin test," you see a noticeable but very slight, well-defined white circle on the processed QA film. This would indicate
   A. Chemical film fog from improper film storage.
   B. Weak or exhausted chemicals.
   C. A light leak around the door or unsafe safelights.
   D. Inadequate exposure time before processing.

10. Given that exposure errors are not the problem, processed films that are too dark may be the result of
    A. Underdevelopment or weak developer.
    B. Overdevelopment or overly warm temperature.
    C. Underfixation or weak fixer.
    D. Overfixation or overly warm fixer.
    E. None of the above.

11. An overall graying of the film, decreasing diagnostic usability, could result from which of the following?
    A. A light leak around the door.
    B. Excessive wattage of the bulb in the safelight.
    C. Safelight too close to the working area.
    D. A crack in the safelight filter.
    E. All of the above.
12. The primary reason that automatic processors are much faster than manual processing is that
    A. Automatic processors have lower developing temperatures.
    B. Automatic processors have higher developing temperatures.
    C. Automatic processors skip the rinse cycle.
    D. Automatic processors have rollers that act as squeegees.
13. You remove from a patient's chart radiographs that are now 2 years old. They appear rather brownish and opaque, making interpretation difficult at best. This could be caused by all of the following except
    A. Inadequate washing time.
    B. Overdevelopment.
    C. Inadequate fixing time.
    D. Exhausted fixer.
14. The reducing agent in the developer responsible for building the black and gray tones is
    A. Potassium bromide.
    B. Metol or hydroquinone.
    C. Ammonium thiosulfate.
    D. Sodium carbonate.
15. The fixing agent that clears the unexposed crystals is
    A. Acetic or sulfuric acid.
    B. Sodium sulfite.
    C. Ammonium thiosulfate.
    D. Aluminum chloride or sulfide.

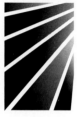

Chapter 3

X-Ray Properties and the Generation of X Rays

INTRODUCTION

The first two chapters taught basic techniques of radiographic imaging. But how did the "magic" happen? How were the x rays produced? What properties do they possess that allow them to record the patient's image on the film? We'll begin with the discovery of x rays.

Wilhelm Conrad Roentgen (1845–1925), a Bavarian physicist, was experimenting with Hittorf-Crookes tubes. These sealed glass tubes were partially evacuated, leaving only small amounts of air inside. Each tube contained cathode and an anode. When Roentgen applied high-voltage currents to one of these tubes, he noticed that a fluorescent screen near the tube glowed. Roentgen placed various materials, including his own hand, between the tube and the screen to determine if the "rays" coming from the tube could be obstructed. The resulting image of his hand bones on the fluorescent screen changed medical history. Roentgen had discovered x rays on November 8, 1895.

PROPERTIES OF X RAYS

X rays themselves are not unique. They are part of a spectrum of electromagnetic radiation, some rays of which are visible and some invisible (Fig. 3–1). However, x rays have technique properties that make them especially useful in medicine and dentistry. X rays can

1. *Penetrate* matter.
2. Produce a *latent image.*
3. Produce *fluorescence* in certain materials.
4. Produce *ionization* of substances (matter).

The remainder of this chapter discusses the properties of x-ray *penetration* and *ionization.* The production of a latent image and the production of screen fluorescence by x rays are discussed in other chapters.

"Particulate" Radiation

X rays are "packets" of energy that travel, with properties both of waves (electromagnetic radiation) and of particles. An x ray as a particle or bundle of energy is termed an x-ray photon. The x-ray photon has no mass or charge and moves in straight lines at the speed of light (186,000 miles per second). These x-ray photons interact with electrons in the x-ray tube, in the patient, and on the x-ray film.

Interactions of x rays with the electrons within the tubehead or the patient are called ionizations. *Ionization* is the process whereby electrons are removed from

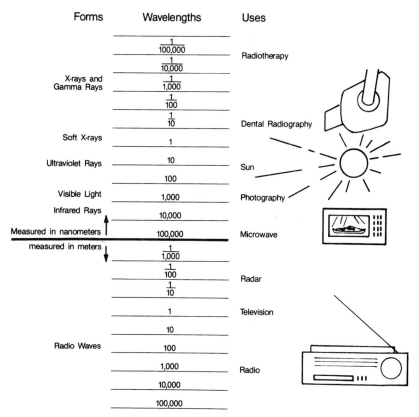

Figure 3–1. Electromagnetic spectrum showing the various wavelengths of commonly employed radiations.

atoms through collisions with x-ray photons. The atoms that lose electrons become positive ions. Both the positive ions (ionized atoms) and the negative ions (electrons) are unstable structures. The electrons ejected from the atom can speed off to interact with other atoms, tissues, or chemicals. The positive ions can also interact but usually return to a stable state. The importance of the process of ionization is discussed in Chapter 13. This chapter explains how x rays are produced by collisions of high-speed electrons with a metal "target" in the dental x-ray tube. The physics of such interactions is termed quantum physics or quantum theory, the discussion of which is beyond the scope of this book. However, some basic interactions that produce the types of radiation called *bremsstrahlung radiation* and *characteristic radiation* are described here.

Bremsstrahlung Radiation

Bremsstrahlung radiation is produced when an electron passes near the nucleus of an atom. The negatively charged (−) electron is deflected by the positively charged (+) nucleus. The energy lost by the deceleration of the electron is emitted in the form of a photon of radiation called bremsstrahlung (from the German word for *braking*) radiation. This process is diagrammed in Figure 3–2. Braking radiation is produced primarily in the dental x-ray tubehead.

Characteristic Radiation

Characteristic radiation results when an electron within an atom is ejected from the inner orbit of the atom by an incoming high-speed electron. With the loss of the electron from the inner orbit, the atom becomes very unstable (and positively charged, or ionized). The vacancy left by the ejected electron is soon filled by an electron from an outer orbit. As this new electron "drops down" into the inner orbit, some of its energy is emitted as a specific x radiation called *characteristic radiation*. This radiation is specific to, or characteristic of the particular atom in which the interaction occurred. Each element emits a particular characteristic energy when its atoms are so bombarded. This process is diagrammed in Figure 3–3.

Characteristic radiation makes up only a small portion of the x rays produced in a dental x-ray unit. However, a process similar to the production of characteristic radiation occurs when x-ray photons interact with a patient's tissues. The incoming x-ray photon ejects an electron from its orbit in a patient's molecule, another electron fills the vacancy, and radiation is emitted from the patient. The interaction of patient tissues and x radiation is presented in more detail in Chapter 13.

Electromagnetic Radiation

Examples of electromagnetic waves or radiation are radiowaves, microwaves, cosmic rays, and visible light. Visible light is a spectrum of colored rays with

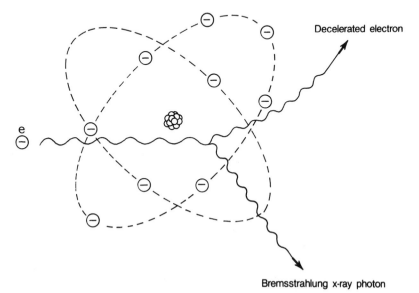

Figure 3–2. Bremsstrahlung radiation. This radiation occurs in the target anode material. The incoming electron (from the cathode) slows as it is drawn to the nucleus of the atom. Some of the energy lost in the deceleration is emitted as an x-ray photon with energy equal to that lost by the electron.

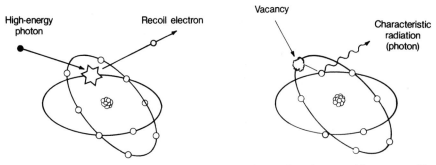

Figure 3–3. The incoming x-ray electron ejects an *inner* electron from the atom; this vacant position is then filled by an *outer* electron. Energy "left over" by the difference between these two electrons is "given off" as characteristic radiation with an energy specific to the atom bombarded.

different wavelengths. The visible rays are those seen in the colors of a rainbow; the invisible rays are *ultraviolet* (*above* our eyes' range) and *infrared* (*below* our eyes' range). X rays, too, are an invisible spectrum of rays or radiation with different wavelengths. Each type of x ray in this spectrum has its *characteristic wavelength,* which determines the frequency of the waves. The shorter the wavelength—that is, the more waves that pass a particular point in a given time—the higher the wave frequency. High-frequency, short-wavelength x rays are more penetrating, and low-frequency, long-wavelength x rays are less penetrating. Figure 3–4 shows two x rays with different wavelengths and frequencies. The shorter wavelength radiation (*b*) is more penetrating than the longer (*a*). An x ray is made more or less penetrating in a dental tube by the selection of a high or low kilovoltage (kV).

Kilovoltage (kV)

A *volt (V)* is a unit of electrical potential that can be considered a measure of work capacity. In an electrical system, the potential difference between a negatively and a positively charged pole creates an electrical "pressure." The greater the

a
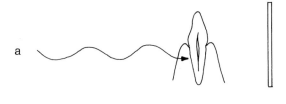

b
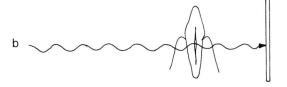

Figure 3–4. X ray *a* has a long wavelength; that is, the distance between its peaks is greater than for x ray *b*. It is therefore less penetrating and will usually be stopped within the object it enters, depositing its energy in that object. X ray *b* has a shorter wavelength and is therefore more penetrating; it proceeds through the material to strike the x-ray film and registers a portion of the image of that object.

electrical potential, the more pressure or potential energy is in the system. Higher voltages mean greater energies. Household voltage is 110 V; x-ray units often require 220 V.

The x-ray machine converts 220 V to the several thousand volts needed to generate x rays by means of a step-up transformer. A transformer is an electromagnetic device that changes current from low to high voltage or vice versa. A step-up transformer raises the voltage, whereas a step-down transformer lowers it (Fig. 3–5). The electrical potential between the *cathode* (negative side) and *anode* (positive side) in an x-ray unit is increased to such a high level that it is measured in *kilovolts (kV)* rather than volts. A kilovolt equals 1,000 volts. Some dental x-ray machines allow the operator to select a kilovoltage peak (kVp), or maximum, setting in the range of 50 to 100 kV. Other units have predetermined kilovolt peak settings: 70 and 90 kVp are the most common.

A higher kilovolt peak setting will produce x-rays that are more energetic, have greater penetrating power, and have a greater capacity to pass through matter. Low-energy x rays tend to be absorbed by the matter through which they pass, including body tissues. If the x rays are absorbed by the patient, they will not reach the radiographic film to make an image. Therefore, kilovoltages lower than 65 kVp are rarely used in dentistry. The amount of energy in an x-ray beam is sometimes referred to as the *quality* of the beam. **The kVp setting on the x-ray machine influences the quality, or energy, of the x rays produced.**

As mentioned, the two common settings for dental x-ray machines are 70 kVp and 90 kVp. For every 15 percent increase in kilovoltage, the density on the resulting radiograph will double. Although 15 kV is a little more than 15 percent of 70 or 90 kV, a "15 kV" rule works well as a baseline. Going from 70 kV to 85 kV essentially doubles the density of the film. Stated another way, increasing the kilovoltage by 15 requires decreasing the time by one-half to keep the same radiographic density. Conversely, decreasing the kilovoltage by 15 requires doubling the time to keep the same radiographic density.

Milliamperage (mA)

An *ampere (A)* is the unit of electrical current, or the number of electrons flowing, in an electrical circuit. The amount of current needed in an x-ray machine

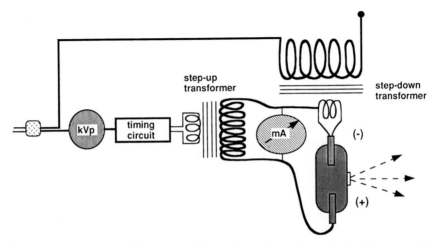

Figure 3–5. Extremely simplified diagram of the circuitry and transformers involved in x-ray production.

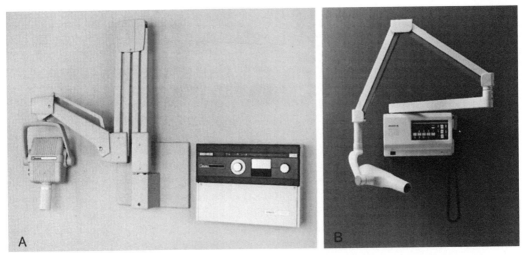

Figure 3–6. *A,* Traditional control panel with milliamperage selector, kilovoltage-peak selector, and exposure-time selector. The panel is capable of controlling as many as three different x-ray machines. *B,* More contemporary control panel. Milliamperage and kilovoltage peak are predetermined, and selecting a facsimile of the tooth to be imaged automatically determines the time of exposure. (Courtesy of the Belmont Corporation, Somerset, NJ.)

is low, and the amperage is measured in *milliamperes (mA)*, or 1/1,000 ampere. Some dental x-ray units offer a choice of milliampere settings: usually 10 and 15 mA. Other dental x-ray units may have a predetermined single milliampere setting, perhaps as low as 6 or 7 mA.

The current in the filament circuit in an x-ray machine is used to heat a very thin wire (a *filament*) made of tungsten. Heating the filament "agitates" the tungsten atoms; some of the electrons in these atoms escape from their orbits. This action, called *thermionic emission,* can be thought of as a "boiling off" of tungsten electrons. Although the process is different, think of the concept as similar to water molecules escaping as steam from boiling water. The tungsten electrons that have been "boiled off" form a cloud around the filament, and it is these "free" electrons that are ultimately responsible for generating x rays.

As a greater amount of current is applied to the filament, more heat is generated and more electrons are "boiled off." **The milliampere setting in the x-ray unit influences the current flowing through the filament and therefore the number, or** *quantity,* **of x rays that will be produced in the x-ray tube.** The other factor that influences the number of x rays produced is the length of exposure time. In some dental x-ray units, the time of exposure is the only factor within the operator's control (Fig. 3–6).

COMPONENTS OF A DENTAL X-RAY TUBE

Cathode

The cathode is the negatively charged end of an x-ray tube. In a dental x-ray tube, the cathode consists of the tungsten filament and a focusing cup (Fig. 3–7).

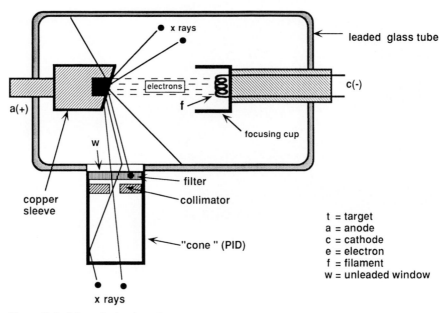

Figure 3–7. Schematic drawing of a conventional dental x-ray tube. The x rays are represented as photons (bundles or packets of energy). The leaded glass does not permit many x rays to exit the tube. In fact, most of the x rays are absorbed by the leaded glass. The photons that are used for diagnosis escape the tube through the unleaded window.

Focusing Cup

The focusing cup has a negative electrostatic charge and is usually made of molybdenum. The shape of the cup and its negative charge repel the electrons (also negatively charged) coming from the filament and keep them suspended in a "cloud" around the filament. When the high-voltage circuit is activated, the focusing cup's charge and shape help direct the electrons toward the anode and prevent them from spreading out and missing their target.

Anode

The anode, the positive end of the x-ray tube, is made of tungsten and copper. A small block of tungsten is embedded in a larger copper stem or sleeve to act as the *target* for the electrons. Tungsten is used because it has a high atomic number and thus can produce many x rays. In addition, tungsten has a high melting point (remember the heat produced) and a low vapor pressure. It will not melt, or vaporize, unless extremely long exposures are made or unless many exposures are made in a short period of time. Copper is used around the tungsten target to conduct heat rapidly away from the target, thus reducing the wear by heat on the target.

Filter

In most dental x-ray tubes, an aluminum filter in the form of a disc is placed at the port, or opening, of the open-ended cylinder (Fig. 3–8). The small fraction of

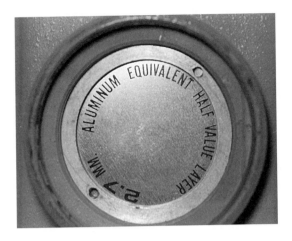

Figure 3–8. This photograph shows the added filtration—an aluminum disc placed near the exit on part of the tubehead. The cone has been removed for illustration.

x rays that is allowed to escape (1 percent) must pass through this filter. Many of the lower-energy x rays, those with long wavelengths, are prevented from reaching the patient or the film by this added filter. By law, dental x-ray machines operating below 70 kV must have 1.5 mm of added aluminum filtration. Those with a kilovolt peak of 70 or above must have 2.5 mm of aluminum filtration. The additional filtration required for the higher kilovolt machines is necessary because of the higher average energy (mean energy) of the x rays produced in these machines. The filtration is necessary to remove low-energy x rays, which add to the absorbed dose in the patient's skin but which may not reach the film.

Tubehead Housing

All the structures discussed so far are surrounded by a glass envelope in a vacuum environment. The glass envelope, in turn, is housed by metal (usually lead). The metal insulates the tubehead components and reduces the amount of radiation that can "leak" from the tubehead housing.

Oil

Within the tubehead, the glass tube is immersed in oil to help absorb the heat created by x-ray production (Fig. 3–9). X-ray production is very inefficient, with 99 percent of the energy used to generate x rays being lost as heat.

Collimator

The collimator is a disc of metal, usually lead, that has a small aperture that restricts the size or shape of the x-ray beam as it exits the tubehead (Fig. 3–10). Thus, collimation is the restriction of the x-ray beam size by a lead diaphragm. According to federal regulation, the diameter of the restricted beam must not exceed 2¾ inches (7 cm) at the patient's skin surface.

Lead-lined "cones" or cylinders effect a second collimation of the x-ray beam. Figure 3–11A shows an example of a standard, open-ended cylinder. This cylinder

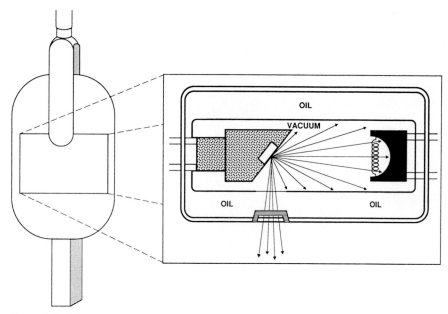

Figure 3–9. Schematic drawing of a conventional dental x-ray tubehead. The tube is immersed in oil to help dissipate the heat produced during the generation of x rays.

further directs the x-ray beam to the area of interest. More recently, manufacturers have introduced rectangular collimating devices (Figs. 3–11B and 3–12) that reduce the beam size even more and consequently reduce the skin surface area exposed to x radiation. The description of the technique in Chapter 1 using the paralleling instruments included examples of rectangular collimation. Figure 3–13 illustrates the dramatic reduction in skin surface area exposed to the beam when a rectangular cone is used.

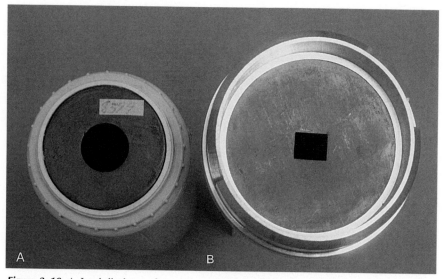

Figure 3–10. *A,* Lead diaphragm for round, open-ended cylinder. *B,* Lead diaphragm for rectangular cylinder.

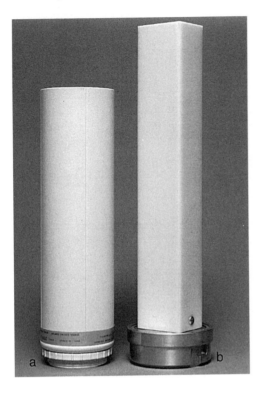

Figure 3–11. *A,* standard round, open-ended, lead-lined cylinder. *B,* Rectangular, open-ended, lead-lined cone or cylinder.

PRODUCTION OF X RAYS

Following is a step-by-step explanation of the way x rays are produced in an x-ray tube. Although it seems like a long and complicated process, it occurs instantaneously when the exposure button is pressed. You may want to refer to Figure 3-7 for a review of the dental x-ray tube components.

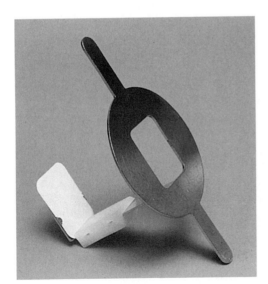

Figure 3–12. A position-indicating device that may be used with open-ended, round cylinders to further collimate the x-ray beam.

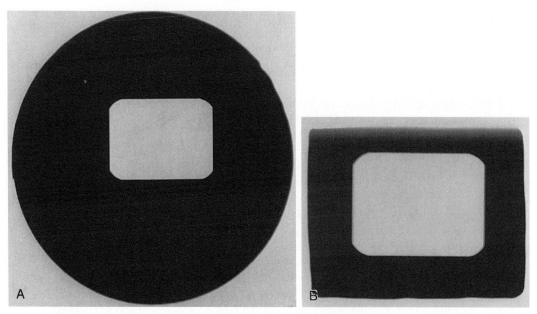

Figure 3–13. *A,* The round area represents the amount of skin surface that would be exposed using a round, open-ended cylinder. *B,* The skin surface area exposed using rectangular position-indicating devices.

- The operator turns on the x-ray machine.
- The operator selects the kilovoltage peak and millampere settings, if appropriate.
- The operator selects the exposure time. The exposure time is the length of time the x rays are actually produced. In dental units, this time is usually less than 1 second.
- The operator presses the exposure button.
- Electrical current passing through the filament "boils off" electrons through thermionic emission.
- The potential difference between the cathode (negatively charged side) and the anode (positively charged side) of the tube is activated. The electrons, which have a negative charge, are attracted to the positive anode at extremely high speeds. Nothing impedes their progress because the x-ray tube is a vacuum tube: there are no air molecules inside it.
- The electrons from the filament collide with the *target* at the anode end of the tube. The collision of the high-speed electrons against the target produces energy in the form of x rays.
- X rays are generated in all directions (360°) from the target. The x rays travel at the speed of light.
- Most of the x rays produced are absorbed by the leaded glass x-ray tube and the metal housing surrounding the x-ray tube.
- A small portion of the x rays generated escape the x-ray tube through an unleaded area in the glass, the *window.*
- These escaped x rays then pass through a *filter,* which absorbs the less useful, lower-energy x rays in the beam.
- The x-ray beam then passes through a lead *collimator,* which restricts the spread of the beam. The x rays that pass through the opening in the collimator (the *port*) travel through the x-ray cone to reach the patient and image receptor.

Study Questions

1. Which of the following is not a characteristic of an x ray?
   A. It travels with a wave-like motion.
   B. It travels at 186,000 miles per second in a vacuum.
   C. It causes ionization in matter.
   D. It has a mass equal to its density.

2. Which of the following statements is false?
   A. X-ray photons with the highest energy have the shortest wavelengths.
   B. The kilovoltage determines the energy or penetrating power of the x ray.
   C. Changing the milliamperage alters the wavelengths of the x ray.
   D. The amount of electrons released in the "boiling off" process affects the number of x-ray photons produced.

3. A beam that is properly collimated should
   A. Pass through a 1.5-mm aluminum disc at the exit or portal.
   B. Pass through a 2.5-mm aluminum disc at the exit or portal.
   C. Be restricted to a diameter of 2 inches at the skin.
   D. Be restricted to a diameter of 234 inches at the skin.

4. An x-ray photon is
   A. A small particle able to penetrate matter.
   B. A small bundle of pure energy with wave-like and particle-like properties.
   C. An electron that has been accelerated to 186,000 miles per second.
   D. An electrical current that has been magnified by 1000 V or 1 kV.

5. X rays are actually produced in the tube by
   A. Radioactive decay of particulate matter.
   B. Electrical current passing through a mixture of oil and gases, creating minute explosions.
   C. High-speed electrons colliding with the electrons in the target, giving off radiation.
   D. High-speed photons colliding with the electrons in the oil mixture and target area.

6. What percent of the energy generated by the collision between electrons from the cathode and the anode is actually converted to x radiation?
   A. 99 percent.
   B. 10 percent.
   C. 2 percent.
   D. 1 percent.

7. The term *thermionic emission* refers to
   A. The heating of the tungsten filament to such a degree that the electrons "boil off" and form a cloud around the filament.
   B. The excessive production of heat that occurs during x-ray generation.
   C. The ability of the x rays emitted from the x-ray tube to produce reddening of the skin when an overexposure occurs.
   D. The radioactive contamination that is produced but contained within the x-ray tube during x-ray generation.

8. The unit of measure for the amount of electricity that flows through an electrical wire is the
   A. Ampere.
   B. Volt.

C. Watt.

D. Hertz.

9. The difference between the negative side and the positive side of the x-ray tube creates an attraction. The greater the difference is, the greater the attraction. The greater the attraction is, the greater the speed of the electrons flying from one side of the tube to the other. The greater the speed is, the greater the impact upon collision. This description refers to the effect of changing the

A. Milliamperage.

B. Exposure time.

C. Kilovoltage.

D. Thickness of filtration.

10. If a machine could produce 10,000 x-ray photons in 1 second, but you wanted it to produce more than that, what would you change to get the greatest increase?

A. The milliamperage.

B. The exposure time.

C. The kilovoltage.

D. The thickness of filtration.

11. Filtration is used to

A. Remove excessive amounts of radiation.

B. Narrow the beam to a specified diameter.

C. Absorb excessive heat during production.

D. Remove long-wavelength x-ray photons.

12. The anode contains the

A. Positively charged target and is where primary x-ray production takes place.

B. Positively charged target and is where the electrons are released during thermionic emission.

C. Negatively charged target and is where primary x-ray production takes place.

D. Negatively charged target and is where the electrons are released during thermionic emission.

E. Positively charged filament and is where the electrons are released during thermionic emission.

F. Negatively charged filament and is where primary x-ray production takes place.

13. Just as a car at high speed "brakes," or loses some of its speed (energy) as it turns a sharp corner, so does a high-speed electron. With the electron, the energy "lost" is not really lost, but transferred to another form: an x-ray photon. This phenomenon is called

A. Characteristic radiation.

B. Radioactive decay.

C. Particulate gamma radiation.

D. Bremsstrahlung radiation.

14. Most of the energy during x-ray generation is transferred from kinetic energy (the high-speed electrons) to energy in the form of

A. X-ray photons.

B. Heat.

C. Gamma radiation.

D. Radioactive decay.

Chapter 4

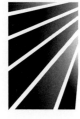

Image Characteristics

Up to this point you have learned how to position, expose, and process a radiograph. You have discovered some of the properties of x rays and how x rays interact with matter, the patient, and the film emulsion. You know how x rays are generated in the dental x-ray tube. You have produced your first radiographs.

How do you judge the quality of your radiograph? What does a "good" radiograph look like? What are the image characteristics that constitute a diagnostically useful radiograph?

In the next few chapters, we answer these questions. We describe film qualities, patient factors, and technical and processing errors that directly affect the image and film quality. This chapter describes the visual characteristics (film qualities) of the x-ray image that make a film diagnostically useful. These image characteristics are outlined in Table 4–1.

VISUAL QUALITIES OF AN X-RAY IMAGE

Contrast

An x ray is basically a black and white picture but one that includes multiple shades of gray. The darkest area of the x ray is black, the lightest, white. In radiologic terms, *black* is referred to as *radiolucent* and *white* as *radiopaque*. Figure 4–1 is a bitewing radiograph. The white area marked *a* is a silver filling (an amalgam). The dark area, *b*, represents air and soft tissue of the cheek. Because the x rays pass through the cheek and expose a lot of film emulsion (recall Chapter 2), this area is black. On the other hand, the x rays are stopped completely by the silver filling; no emulsion is exposed, and thus no image is recorded—this area is white. These two regions of the film highly *contrast* with each other: one is black and one is white.

Contrast is also defined as the difference between the "shades of gray," or densities. The overall contrast on a radiograph is the product of both the film contrast and the subject contrast. Except for choosing the type of film to use, the clinician has little control over film contrast. Furthermore, as we have seen earlier, attenuation, or stopping, of x rays in an object or patient also affects the contrast of a film. Although we can do nothing to change patients' thickness or tissue differences, we *can* alter the kilovoltage (kV) and/or the mAs (milliamperage × time in seconds) to compensate for patient differences.

TABLE 4–1. IMAGE CHARACTERISTICS

VISUAL CHARACTERISTICS	GEOMETRIC CHARACTERISTICS
Contrast	Unsharpness/magnification
Film	Geometric
Subject	Motion
Density	Distortion
Detail	

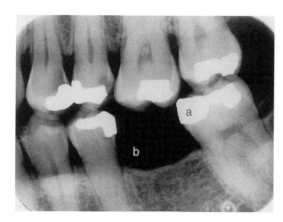

Figure 4–1. Bitewing radiograph. The white area (*a*) is an amalgam, and the dark area (*b*) represents air and soft tissue of the cheek.

Film Contrast

Film contrast depends on three things: (1) the type of film; (2) the processing of the film; and (3) the density of the film. The film type applies primarily to extraoral x-ray films. Each film type has its own inherent contrast; each is evaluated by a test called a characteristic curve. The discussion of this test can be found in other dental radiography texts.

Film processing, as described in Chapter 2, can also influence the contrast of a film. A developing time that is too long will darken the film, and the subtle shades of gray will be lost; the overall image will be uniformly dark (Fig. 4–2). Similarly, underprocessing, either because of insufficient time or low temperature, will decrease film contrast. The underprocessed film will be uniformly light and gray (Fig. 4–3). Again, the different shades (contrast) are lost.

The degree of darkness or lightness of a film is called the *film density.* Some clinicians like dark films, and others, less dark. The correct density of a film should enable the observer to view the grays of soft tissues and bone as well as the blacks and whites of airways and fillings (Fig. 4–4) (see the discussion of density later in this chapter).

Subject Contrast

Obviously, patients are not all alike. Each one has a different height, weight, bone structure, and so on. Even if the same exposure factors are used, an x ray

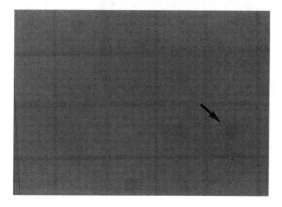

Figure 4–2. Darkened film. Details, seen here as dots, are still visible, but there is little contrast. The *arrow* indicates one of the dots. This film is too dense because of a too-long development time. Compare this with Figure 4–3.

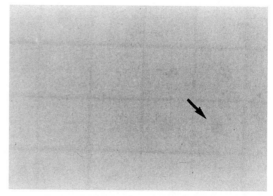

Figure 4–3. This film is uniformly gray or light. Contrast is lost in this image. The dot labeled with the *arrow* is barely visible. This film has insufficient density owing to under-processing or to insufficient development time or temperature.

taken of a child will be very different from that of a 200-lb adult. The *subject contrast* depends on (1) the thickness of the subject; (2) the density of the subject; (3) the atomic number of the tissue of the subject; and (4) the kilovoltage used. On many x-ray units, the operator can adjust only the *kilovoltage* or the *time.* Changing the time will change only the number, or *quantity,* of x rays. Changing the kilovoltage will alter the penetrability, or *quality,* of the x rays, making them better able to pass through tissues. Therefore, kilovoltage is the only exposure parameter over which the operator has control that directly affects subject contrast. Exposure time and milliamperage control only the number of x rays and thus have most of their impact on the density rather than on the contrast of the film image.

Density

As you can see from the previous discussion, contrast and density cannot be readily separated. Contrast is really the difference between densities. *Radiographic density* refers to the degree of "darkness" of an x ray. This density depends on several things, including (1) the amount of radiation reaching the film—either the quantity (mAs) or the quality (kV) of the radiation; (2) the distance from the x-ray tube to the patient; (3) the patient (subject) thickness; and (4) the developing conditions.

Figure 4–4. Black areas between teeth represent soft tissue such as the cheek or gingiva. Dense white areas are restorations. Note the distinct density difference between the enamel, dentin, and pulpal tissues. (See also Chapter 12 for normal anatomy.)

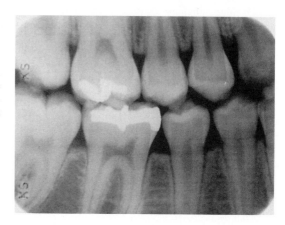

Amount of Radiation

The amount of radiation reaching the film depends on the quantity of photons produced and their opportunity to reach the image receptor. The more x-ray photons that strike the film, the more dense, or black, is the radiograph. Recall from Chapter 3 that the milliamperage influences the number of x rays produced in an x-ray tube, and that longer exposure times allow more x rays to reach the film. The product of the milliamperage and the time of exposure in seconds is expressed as *mAs*. This product has the greatest impact on the quantity of radiation produced.

If two films are to have the same density, they should have the same mAs product. If other factors are constant, an exposure made at 10 mA and 0.3 second will produce the same density as one made at 15 mA and 0.2 second:

$$10 \text{ mA} \times 0.3 \text{ sec} = 3 \text{ mAs}$$

$$15 \text{ mA} \times 0.2 \text{ sec} = 3 \text{ mAs}$$

The kilovoltage peak (kVp) also influences the amount of radiation reaching the film. The higher the kilovoltage peak, the more energy the beam will have and the greater will be its penetrating power. A greater penetrating power means that more x rays will pass through the patient and reach the film rather than being absorbed by the patient's tissues. If you increase the kilovoltage peak by 15 kV, you must decrease the exposure time by half to keep the densities of the films similar. If you decrease the kilovoltage peak by 15 kV, you must double the time of exposure to maintain similar densities. For example, if you produce one film at 75 kVp and 0.5 second, and you want to produce a second film at 90 kVp, you must reduce the exposure time of the second film to 0.25 second to have similar densities on the two films. On the other hand, if you produce one film at 85 kVp and 0.3 second and you want to produce a second film at 70 kVp, you must increase the exposure time for the second film to 0.6 second.

Distance the X Rays Travel

The distance the x rays travel is called the *source* (x-ray tube)-*to-film distance* (SFD). The intensity (and thus the degree of darkness or density) of the x-ray beam varies inversely as the square of the distance from the source. This is called the **inverse square law** and is written

$$I = \frac{1}{d^2}$$

where I = intensity (density) and d = distance.

A simple formula will help calculate the new exposure times to use if you change the SFD—for instance, from an 8-inch to a 16-inch cylinder.

$$\frac{I_1}{I_2} = \frac{(d_2)^2}{(d_1)^2}$$

The farther away one moves the x-ray tube or source, the less intense the x-ray beam becomes. Therefore, in order to maintain the same radiographic density, you must increase the *exposure time* accordingly. Figure 4–5 illustrates this concept. **Example:** One exposure is made at 8 inches using 0.4 second. When the tubehead is moved to 16 inches away, the intensity (I) will be one-fourth as much, because we doubled the distance (d) from 8 to 16 inches:

$$I = \frac{1}{(2)^2}$$

Consequently, we would have to increase our exposure time by a factor of 4 (4 × 0.4 seconds) to 1.6 seconds in order to maintain the same film density. Using our formula, this would be

$$\frac{I_1}{I_2} = \frac{(d_2)^2}{(d_1)^2}$$

or

$$\frac{0.4}{x} = \frac{(16)^2}{(8)^2}$$

$$x = (0.4 \times 4)$$

$$x = 1.6$$

In summary, to paraphrase the inverse square law: whatever change you make to the distance, square it, and make the same change to the time.

Scale of Contrast

The x-ray film's *range of useful densities* is its scale of contrast. If a radiographic film is black and white, it has only two useful densities and thus has a *short contrast scale*. If a radiographic film has many shades of gray, including black and white, then it has a *long contrast scale*. In general, high-kilovoltage techniques have a longer scale of contrast, with more shades of gray, or more useful densities, on the film. Low-kilovoltage techniques (65 kV or less) have short contrast scales—only blacks and whites. Figure 4–6 shows a comparison of short- and long-scale radiographic contrasts. Some extraoral films are manufactured for high contrast (short contrast scale) and some for less contrast (long contrast scale.)

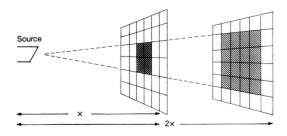

Figure 4–5. Using our formula, $I = I/d^2$, we can make a ratio of the "original" intensity, I_o, to the "new" intensity, I_n, which can be written where d_o is the "original" distance, and d_n is the "new" distance.
$I_o/I_n = (d_n)^2/(d_o)^2$

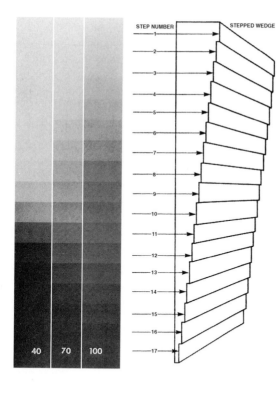

Figure 4–6. Radiographs taken at 40kV are predominantly black and white; that is, they have high contrast (a short contrast scale). Those taken at 100 kV show many shades of gray (a long contrast scale).

Detail

Film *detail* is also known as *resolution.* An x-ray image has good detail if small objects can be easily identified in the film without distortion, overlap, or unsharpness. The detail or sharpness depends on several things, including (1) the focal spot size, (2) the radiographic contrast, and (3) certain geometric characteristics. In general, intraoral film demonstrates greater detail than extraoral film.

Focal Spot Size

The focal spot size is determined by the size and the angulation of the target anode (see Fig. 12–5). The smaller the focal spot size is, the better the resolution, or detail, of the x-ray image. Figure 4–7 shows a diagram of a conventional dental x-ray tube focal spot. As you can see, the *effective focal spot* can be made smaller than the *actual focal spot* by angling the tungsten target (anode) approximately 20

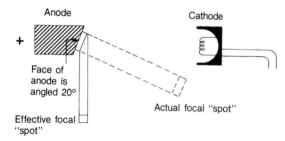

Figure 4–7. The target when viewed from below (where the x rays would exit) appears smaller than viewed from the cathode because of the angulation of the anode. The technique of angling the target anode 20 degrees reduces the size of the effective focal spot and results in better resolution.

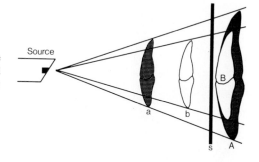

Figure 4–8. Object *a* is farther from the screen (*s*). Its shadow, *A,* is thus enlarged and is bigger than the shadow (*B*) cast by object *b.*

degrees. A typical tungsten anode has an effective focal spot size of about 1 mm. This size is inherent to the machine and cannot be altered.

GEOMETRIC CHARACTERISTICS

Geometric Unsharpness

There is a certain amount of image unsharpness in every radiograph. Casting an image of teeth onto a dental x ray is similar to casting a shadow. If an object is close to the screen, its shadow's size will be close to its actual size. If the object is moved away from the screen (closer to the light source), then its shadow will be magnified. So it is with x-ray imaging; Figure 4–8 helps to illustrate these points.

Even an object such as a tooth, which is placed as close as possible to the film, will have both an umbra (shadow) and a penumbra (area of unsharpness around the shadow) (Fig. 4–9). Placing the object near the film, or *reducing the object-to-film distance* (OFD), helps to reduce geometric distortion or unsharpness by reducing magnification. In addition, *increasing the SFD* reduces magnification. Finally, having the object and film *parallel* and the central ray or x-ray beam

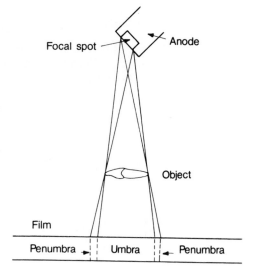

Figure 4–9. Umbra and penumbra cast by the object. The larger the object-film distance is, the greater the penumbra. Increasing the source-film distance reduces the object magnification.

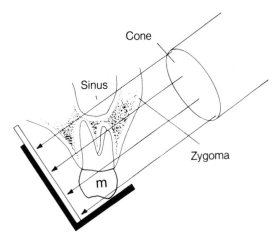

Figure 4–10. In this diagram the long axis of the object, a molar (*m*), is not parallel to the film. Geometric distortion will occur. The image of the molar will be shortened as seen in Figure 4–11.

perpendicular to them also reduces geometric distortion. Figures 4–9 through 4–11 illustrate these concepts.

Motion Unsharpness

Unsharpness caused by patient movement can also be considered a geometric problem. The results of patient movement are seen in Figure 5–27. Some authors still believe that motion unsharpness can be caused by tubehead or x-ray arm movement; but even if the tubehead is vibrating or rocking, there should be no perceptible unsharpness in the x-ray image. *Only* film or patient movement can cause a detectable blurring of the image. Figures 4–12 and 4–13 show images of two paper clips. Both images were exposed using settings of 70 kV and 15 mA for eight impulses (i). An operator, wearing a protective apron and gloves, physically rocked the tubehead during the exposure in Figure 4–13. No blurring of the image appears in either figure. The x-ray photons traveling at the speed of light

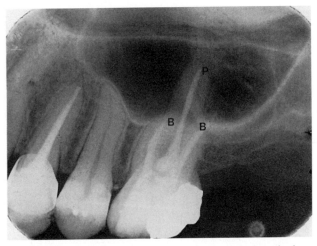

Figure 4–11. See how the buccal roots (*B*) appear far shorter than the palatal root (*P*). Another example of foreshortening is seen is Figure 4–14.

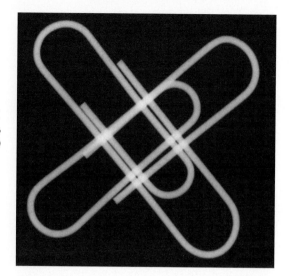

Figure 4–12. X-ray image of two paper clips exposed at settings of 70 kV and 15 mA for eight impulses.

are not altered significantly from their straight-line paths to create motion artifacts. However, movement of the tubehead might spread the photons over a greater surface area of the patient after the photons collide with the cylinder walls.

Distortion

As we have seen, magnification of an x-ray image may result when the OFD is increased. This is a type of distortion. The bisecting-angle technique, because it places the film close to the teeth, *should* minimize this problem. More often, however, this technique is the cause of shape distortion—either elongation or foreshortening. Lines, angles, and long axes of teeth must be visualized or imagined before the correct tube position is guaranteed. More often than not, images like those in Figures 4–14 and 4–15 result. *Shape distortion* resulting from

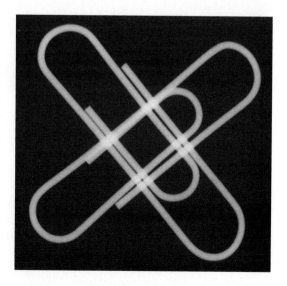

Figure 4–13. Although the operator physically rocked the tubehead during this exposure, the x-ray image of the paper clips does not appear blurred.

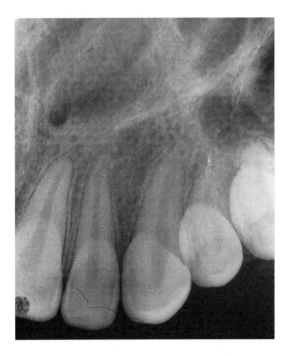

Figure 4–14. Foreshortening.

angulation problems is another image characteristic to avoid. In Figure 4–14, the distortion occurs because the vertical angulation is too steep. In Figure 4–15, the vertical angulation is not steep enough. In Figures 4–10 and 4–11, the distortion occurs because the distance from the object to the film is not equal for all structures—that is, the film is closer to the crowns than to the apices.

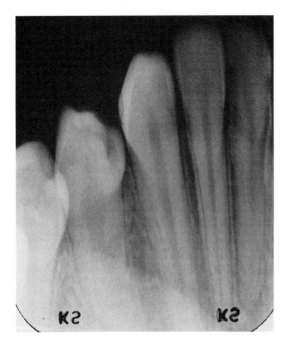

Figure 4–15. Elongation.

Study Questions

1. The term "high contrast" refers to film with
   A. White and black with many shades of gray in between.
   B. White and black with few or no shades of gray in between.
   C. Uniform grayness throughout all aspects of the image.
   D. The characteristic curve created by the variances in the shades of gray.

2. You have processed a film and notice it had poor contrast. In order to correct the problem, you must know all the factors that could influence contrast so that you can check them. Which of the following will not influence contrast?
   A. Developing time may be too long or temperatures too high.
   B. Developing time may be too short or temperatures too low.
   C. The patient was extremely large and the kilovoltage was too low.
   D. The patient moved during x-ray exposure.

3. Radiographic density is a term used to describe
   A. The thickness of the emulsion on the film.
   B. The thickness or density of the subject (i.e., larger patients have more tissue to penetrate).
   C. The degree of darkness or blackness on the film (the overall darkness).
   D. The amount of radiation in the x-ray beam (the density or thickness of the radiation within the beam), which determines how well it will penetrate the subject.

4. Density is affected by
   A. Milliamperage.
   B. Kilovoltage.
   C. Source-to-tube distance.
   D. Proper processing.
   E. All of the above.

5. Each object is projected onto a radiograph with a shadow/umbra (the object itself) and an outline/penumbra. Having a thick or wide outline makes the object appear fuzzy or unsharp. Which of the following would cause a wide outline/penumbra, giving an unsharp image?
   A. Decreasing the source-to-object distance.
   B. Increasing the object-to-film distance.
   C. Patient motion.
   D. All of the above.

6. The intensity of the x-ray beam (which produces darkness on the film) will decrease as the distance from the x-ray tube to the film is increased. This is a description of
   A. Radiographic density.
   B. Subject contrast.
   C. Geometric distortion.
   D. Inverse square law.
   E. None of the above.

   The following questions about this chapter are based on problems/situations/case scenarios. This will test not only your knowledge of the subject material, but also your ability to apply what you have learned.

7. Changing the milliamperage from 10 mA and 30 impulses to 15 mA will require what new exposure time in impulses (i)?

   A. 5 i.
   B. 20 i.
   C. 45 i.
   D. 15 i.

8. A dental office uses an exposure time of 30/60 second at 10 mA. If the milliamperage is increased to 15 mA, what is the new exposure time in seconds?
   A. 1 second.
   B. 42/60 second.
   C. 30/60 second.
   D. 20/60 second.
   E. 10/60 second.

9. You work in a dental practice that uses 70 kV, 60 i, a 16-inch cone or position-indicating device (PID), and 15 mA. The dentist retires, and the new dentist who buys his practice asks you to stay on and work for him. One of the things he changes is the kilovoltage, increasing it from 70 kV to 90 kV. What will you do with the other exposure factors to compensate?
   A. Reduce the exposure time to 30 i.
   B. Reduce the exposure time to 15 i.
   C. Reduce the milliamperage to 10 mA.
   D. Increase the distance.
   E. Increase the exposure time to 45 i.

10. The same dentist asks you to do an occlusal film on one of his patients. To do this, you must change the cylinder (i.e., cone or PID) to a 4-inch cylinder. What do you do with the exposure factors to maintain proper density?
   A. Increase milliamperage to the next highest setting.
   B. Decrease kilovoltage from 90 kV to 70 kV.
   C. Decrease time from 30 i to 15 i.
   D. Decrease time from 30 i to 4 i.
   E. Increase time from 30 i to 60 i.

11. Your current exposure factors are a 16-inch PID, 36 i, 10 mA, and 90 kV. You have a female patient with Parkinson's disease. She can hold the film holder in her mouth quite well, but tremors cause her head to shake just enough to cause blurring on the film. You have both paralleling and bisecting-angle film-holding devices. How can you get a better image?
   A. Increase milliamperage to 15 mA and reduce exposure time to 18 i.
   B. Decrease kilovoltage and reduce exposure time to 18 i.
   C. Decrease the PID to 4 inches, increase milliamperage to 15 mA, and reduce exposure time to 9 i.
   D. Decrease the PID to 8 inches, increase milliamperage to 15 mA, and reduce exposure time to 6 i.

Use the following exposure factors for the next three questions: distance = 16 inches; kilovoltage = 70 kV; milliamperage = 10 mA; time = 60 i.

12. Increasing the kilovoltage to 90 kV will require a new exposure time of
   A. 36 i.
   B. 30 i.
   C. 24 i.
   D. 18 i.
   E. 12 i.

13. Decreasing the distance to 8 inches will require a new exposure time of
    A. 30 i.
    B. 24 i.
    C. 15 i.
    D. 9 i.
    E. 4 i.
14. Increasing the milliamperage to 15 mA will require a new exposure time of
    A. 40 i.
    B. 30 i.
    C. 24 i.
    D. 18 i.
    E. 4 i.

Chapter 5

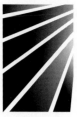

Technique/Processing Errors and Troubleshooting

"There is no shortage of errors."* Errors made during either the exposure phase or the processing phase of intraoral radiography often result in excess exposure to ionizing radiation (x rays) for the patient. Films that are undiagnostic are almost always retaken. Each retake of a dental radiograph *doubles* the absorbed x-ray dose to the patient in that anatomic region.

Learning the most common radiographic errors and their correction during the preclinical phase of your career will save *you* embarrassment and *your patient* unnecessary radiation exposure. Most errors in intraoral radiographic techniques can be divided into two categories: (1) exposure technique and (2) film processing. Before we examine these categories, let us review the criteria for a diagnostically useful intraoral radiograph. Table 5–1 outlines criteria for both the intraoral periapical radiograph and the bitewing radiograph.

ERRORS IN EXPOSURE TECHNIQUE

Mistakes in exposure technique can be subdivided into *operator* and *patient* errors. The majority of exposure technique errors are *caused by the operator*. Table 5–2 outlines the most common errors.

Operator Errors

Improper Film Positioning

The correct placement of the x-ray film is the first and most critical step in good exposure technique. Reviewing the criteria for the correct positioning in each anatomic region, as described in Chapter 1, would be helpful before proceeding in this chapter. You will recall that each film is placed to image specific portions of the teeth and related structures. Three guidelines, if followed closely, will minimize film-positioning errors:

1. The distal surface of the cuspid should be visible in the premolar view.
2. The third molar region should be visible in the molar view.
3. The tooth/teeth of interest should be centered.

Distal Surface of the Cuspid Visible in Premolar View. Figure 5–1 reveals that, in most instances, even the ideal positioning of the film for the maxillary cuspid will result in the overlap of the lingual cusp of the first bicuspid onto the distal aspect of the canine (see diagram of the maxillary cuspid view in the "Paralleling Technique" section of Chapter 1). This overlap is almost unavoidable. Therefore, the distal surface *must* be visualized on each of the premolar periapical

---

*Anonymous—overheard in every diagnostic radiology service in North American dental schools.

TABLE 5–1. CRITERIA FOR A DIAGNOSTICALLY USEFUL RADIOGRAPH

PERIAPICAL RADIOGRAPH
1. The correct anatomic area should be represented.
2. At least 3–4 mm (¼ inch) of alveolar bone should be visible beyond the apex.
3. The image should not be elongated or foreshortened.
4. The radiograph should have acceptable density.
5. The radiograph should be free of film-handling or processing errors.
6. The interproximal contacts should not overlap.
7. There should be no cone cuts.
8. The embossed (raised) dot should appear at the incisal or the occlusal edge.
9. In a complete mouth radiograph series, the apex of each tooth should be visible at least once, preferably twice.

BITEWING RADIOGRAPH
1. The interproximal contacts should not be overlapped from the distal surface of the canine to the mesial surface of the third molar.
2. The crowns of the maxillary and mandibular teeth should be centered in the image from top to bottom.
3. The crest of the alveolar bone should be visible with *no* superimposition of the crowns of the adjacent teeth.
4. The occlusal plane should be as horizontal as possible.

and premolar bitewing views. This visualization is mandatory for the detection of carious lesions on the distal surface of the cuspid. Figure 5–2 shows both the *ideal* and the inadequate cuspid views. "The distal of the cuspid *not* showing" describes one of the most common and most critical positioning errors in intraoral radiographic techniques.

Third Molar Region Visible. You will note that this guideline reads "third molar *region*" and not just "third molar." The absence of the third molar clinically (in the mouth) does not mean that it is *not* present in the bone. Unerupted or impacted third permanent molars (wisdom teeth) are very common. If the adult patient states that the wisdom teeth have not been extracted, you must assume that they are present. The molar view you take should extend far enough past the second permanent molar to include all of the third molar—*even if this means "missing," or ignoring the distal surface of the permanent second bicuspid.* This extended view is especially critical in the mandible, where third molars are frequently horizontally impacted and are often larger than the maxillary third molars. Figure 5–3 illustrates this point.

Tooth/Teeth of Interest Centered. This concept is simple, but it is crucial to good radiographic techniques. With any film-holding device, if you center the film in the biteblock and the tooth of interest on the biteblock, there is little chance of incorrect positioning (assuming that you have assembled the instrument correctly to begin with). **Contacting the biteblock with the biting surfaces of the teeth of interest is critical to correct film placement.** For example, in the case of the

TABLE 5–2. EXPOSURE TECHNIQUE ERRORS

	OPERATOR	PATIENT
Improper film positioning	Improper film-holding instrument assembly	Patient movement
Apical areas missing	Improper tubehead angulation	Film movement
Film bending	Overlapping	
Film backward	Cone cutting	
Improper film selection	Overexposure	
Double exposure	Underexposure	

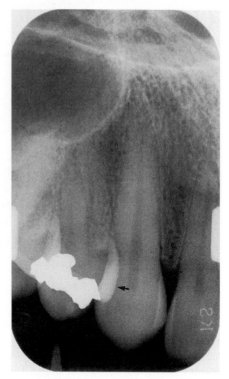

Figure 5–1. Although the maxillary right cuspid is reasonably well centered in the view, the lingual cusp of the first bicuspid is superimposed on the distal contact area of the cuspid (*arrow*). Any interproximal caries could not be detected in this area.

maxillary premolar view, **if we center the bicuspid/molar contact in the middle of the plastic biteblock, the film will normally extend far enough anteriorly to include the cuspid area** (Fig. 5–4).

And, if we center the maxillary or the mandibular second permanent molar in a molar view, we will include all of the third molar region in most cases. Occasionally patient anatomy or tooth position will limit the perfect view. However, if you follow the three guidelines, you will eliminate the positioning errors that are the most common causes of the need to retake films. Other positioning errors are included in the category of "Apical Areas Missing," discussed next.

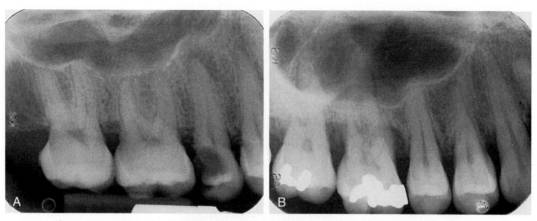

Figure 5–2. A, This view is neither a premolar nor a molar view. It would have missed the distal aspect of the canine or all of the third molar. It demonstrates, therefore, technically incorrect positioning. *B,* This film represents accurate positioning for a maxillary right premolar view.

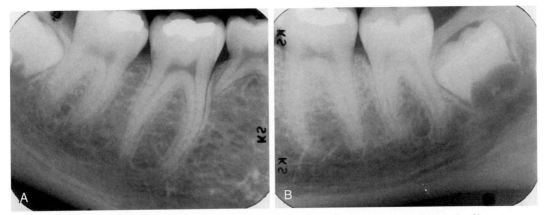

Figure 5–3. *A,* Incorrect positioning—not all of the developing third molar is visible on the film. *B,* Correct positioning.

Apical Areas Missing

One of the most common reasons for the visualization of the apices of the teeth to be missing from the film is that the film was not placed high enough (in the palate) or low enough (in the floor of the mouth) for adequate coverage of the anatomy. With the paralleling technique, when the operator is using positioning instruments, apical areas are missing either because the patient did not close completely or because the biteblock was not contacting the teeth of interest (Fig. 5–5).

Often the latter reason is the cause of the former. If the patient attempts to close while in the position seen in Figure 5–5, the edge of the film will be forced into sensitive tissues; the resulting pain will stop the patient from closing on the film.

Patient anatomy usually dictates the orientation of the long axis of the film. If the floor of the mouth is shallow, perfect parallel placement may be impossible. Any film in any region of the mouth can be angled up to 15 degrees from parallel

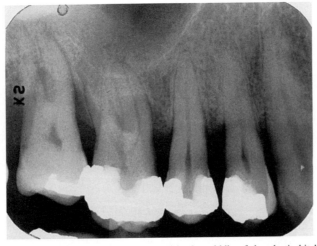

Figure 5–4. If the bicuspid/molar contact is centered in the middle of the plastic biteblock, the film normally extends far enough anteriorly to include the cuspid area.

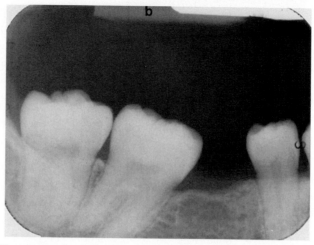

Figure 5–5. The operator placed the biteblock (*b*) at least 1 cm above the occlusal surfaces of the mandibular teeth. The instrument and film may be angled and the tongue gently displaced to allow the biteblock to rest against the teeth of interest *before* the patient closes.

and still be free of significant distortion. Film angles steeper than 15 degrees will cause significant distortion usually in the form of elongation, if the beam is directed perpendicularly to the long axis of the tooth (Fig. 5–6) (see also Chapter 4). Improper tubehead angulation can also cause distortion. Remember, however, that failure to show the root apices in periapical films always necessitates a retake. The operator has complete control over the film placement, including angulation of the film.

Film Bending

Sometimes, to make the patient more comfortable, it is appropriate to *gently* curve, or "bend," the film. This bending allows the film to follow the contours of

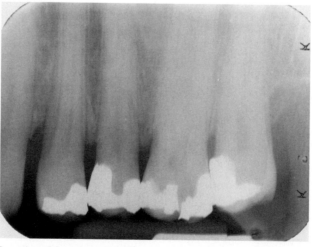

Figure 5–6. Elongation of the apices of maxillary premolars and molars owing to improper angulation (see also Fig. 4–15).

the anatomy more readily (Fig. 5–7*A*). However, gross bending or frank creasing can cause an image distortion (Fig. 5–7*B*) or a crease artifact (labeled *c* in Fig. 5–8).

Note the difference in the image distortion between Figure 5–6 (elongation) and Figure 5–7 (regional distortion). The distortion caused by film bending is localized to the bent region. Distortion owing to elongation is generalized throughout the periapical region.

Placing the Film Backward

The operator must make sure that the sensitive side of the film faces the x-ray tube. If you are in doubt, remember that the back of the film, the side that should *not* face the x-ray source, contains the printed instructions (Figs. 5–9 and 5–10).

Note also in Figure 5–9 that the image of the teeth and surrounding structures is lighter than normal (underexposed) because the lead foil stopped (attenuated) many of the x rays that would have exposed the film and registered the image. Films that have been exposed backward also cause confusion when mounted because the rule regarding the right and left sides of a patient cannot be followed.

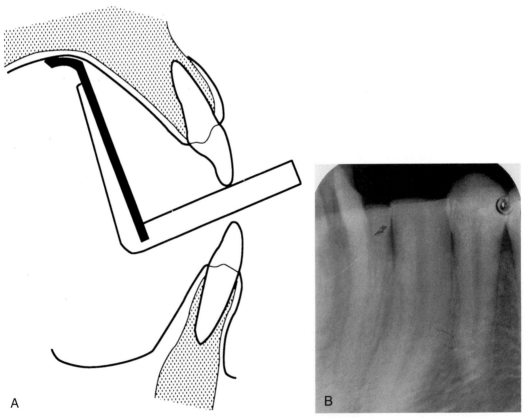

A   B

Figure 5–7. *A* illustrates bending of the upper edge of the film against the palate. Most of the distortion seen in *B* is regional; that is, it occurs where the film was bent in the floor of the mouth. The teeth to the right side of the film are not nearly as distorted.

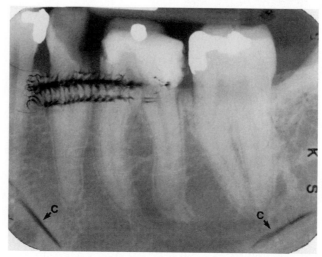

Figure 5–8. The letter *c* designates the crease in the emulsion owing to excessive folding or bending of the film. The artifact, which looks like a "centipede," is due to excessive pressure of a hemostat used to hold the film.

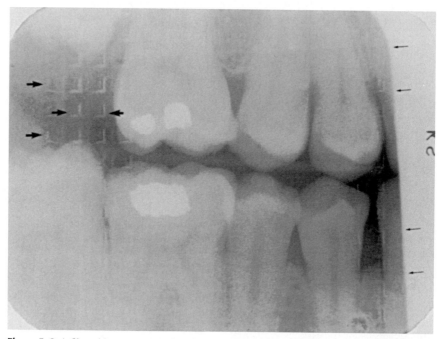

Figure 5–9. A film with many errors. A typical "cone cut" (see also Fig. 5–23) is visible on the right side of the film (*small arrows*). Also present is a "tractor tread," or artifact from the lead foil (*large arrows*), confirming that the film was placed backward.

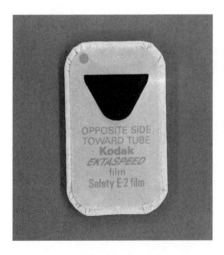

Figure 5–10. Instructions on the back of the film tell the operator which side of the film is to face the x-ray machine.

Improper Film Selection

Chapter 1 showed several examples of different film sizes (see Fig. 1–16). Improper selection of film size will result in many problems. If the film selected is too small, the region or tooth of interest may be missing (Fig. 5–11). If the film selected is too large, the patient will not accept the film comfortably. This discomfort can result in errors of distortion, missed apical areas, patient movement, or overlapping of structures (Figs. 5–12 through 5–15).

The correct film size is one that will adequately cover the area of interest and be comfortable for the patient.

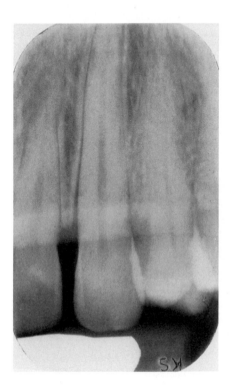

Figure 5–11. A size no. 0 film was selected, and the cuspid apex is missing. A size no. 1 film should have been used.

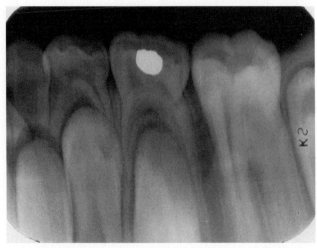

Figure 5–12. Apical areas of primary molars are present but distorted owing to elongation (too shallow a vertical angulation; see also Fig. 5–19).

Double Exposure

You must be careful to separate exposed and unexposed films. Placing into a receptacle the exposed film that you just completed *before* selecting a new film is one way of eliminating double exposures. A film that has been exposed twice will (1) be overexposed, (2) be undiagnostic, and (3) result in a mandatory retake. This usually means that the patient will receive *three times* the necessary radiation dose to the anatomic area that is to be examined. In addition, there is lost time because films have to be retaken. Furthermore, there is embarrassment for you because of the error. Double exposure of films is easily avoided with attention to detail and a systematic approach to placement and exposure.

Improper Instrument Assembly

When preparing film holders that come in separate parts, you should always look through the instrument's indicator ring to ensure that the film is centered in

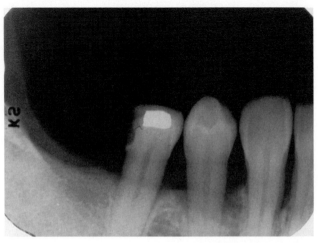

Figure 5–13. Missed apical area. The patient could not tolerate the size no. 2 film and would not close on the instrument.

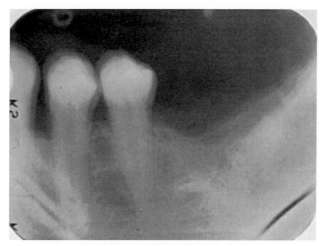

Figure 5–14. The patient moved because the film caused discomfort, leading to motion artifact (blurring). Notice that the operator had bent the film, causing a crease artifact (see also Fig. 5–8).

the ring. If it is not, reassemble the film-holding instrument. Figure 5–16 shows this simple check for proper assembly.

Improper Tubehead (Vertical) Angulation

The proper film has been selected. It is placed correctly in the patient's mouth. The patient is comfortable. Yet various errors could occur subsequent to correct film placement. Aligning the "face" of the tube or cylinder with the indicator ring and paralleling the length of the tube with the indicator rod will ensure the correct vertical tubehead position (Fig. 5–17).

Figures 5–18 and 5–19 show what happens to the radiographic image when the

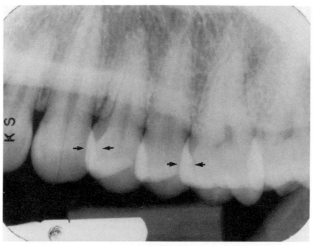

Figure 5–15. Overlapping enamel areas (*arrows*). Here the patient opened slightly and moved the film. The film and instrument were stationary at the time of exposure, but the slight movement of opening shifted the film and changed the horizontal angulation.

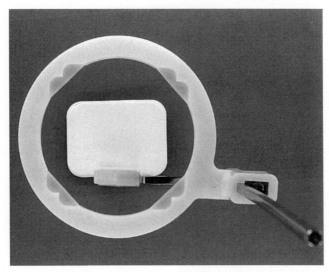

Figure 5–16. Proper instrument assembly.

vertical angulation is too steep—either positively or negatively (causing foreshortening)—or too shallow (causing elongation). Use of the paralleling technique with film-positioning devices minimizes these errors significantly.

Patient anatomy can cause problems also. Knowing a patient's anatomic variations by thoroughly inspecting the patient's mouth clinically will help you reduce the number of undiagnostic radiographs. Figure 5–20A shows a correctly positioned cylinder and film correctly placed in a shallow palate. Note how the film position has changed from a preferred vertical position to a more horizontal one. The film holder is "telling" you to use a very steep vertical angulation, but this would foreshorten the teeth (*arrows,* Fig. 5–20B) and cast the shadow of the zygoma (*z*) onto the teeth apices. Your prior awareness of these potential problems would alert you to "cheat" the instrument—that is, select a slightly more shallow angulation

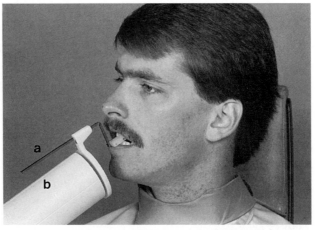

Figure 5–17. The cone is properly aligned with the ring. This proper alignment is confirmed by the orientation of the indicator rod (*a*) parallel to the top of the cylinder and to the indented linear markings (*b*) of the cylinder.

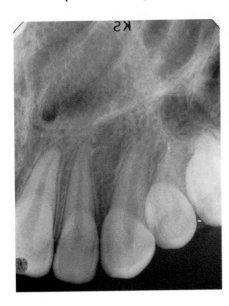

Figure 5–18. Foreshortening.

and thus minimize the potential problems described. *The film holder is an indicating device not a dictating one.*

Overlapping (Improper Horizontal Angulation)

Errors in tube angulation can occur in the horizontal as well as the vertical direction. Improper selection of the horizontal angulation will result in overlapping of interproximal contact areas or approximal enamel surfaces (as in Fig. 5–21A). This error is especially critical in interproximal bitewing radiography. Because many periapical views also afford the clinician another look at carious lesions and

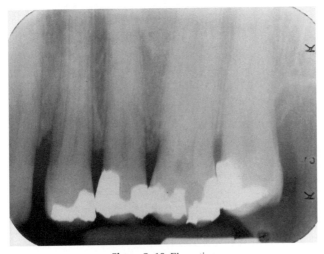

Figure 5–19. Elongation.

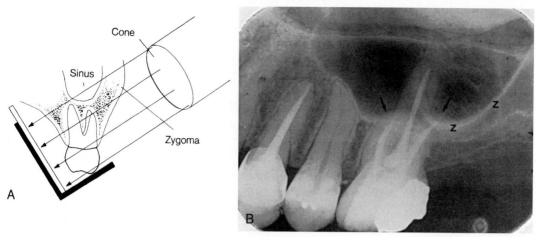

Figure 5–20. *A,* Despite proper instrument placement, the zygoma will be superimposed on the roots. *B,* Foreshortened image.

periodontal bone levels, the operator should always try to open contacts (as in Fig. 5–21*B*) on these views as well.

It is generally accepted that two bitewing views, a premolar and a molar, are necessary to demonstrate correctly all contact areas when the patient has a complete adult dentition (i.e., has third molars). This is because the arch curvature from cuspid to third molar rarely allows one film to demonstrate open contacts of the entire region (Fig. 5–22). For this reason we discourage the use of the no. 3 size bitewing film and suggest that two no. 2 size films are usually necessary to adequately open all contact areas.

Cone Cutting

The term *cone cutting* has stuck with us. The "cone" is really an open-ended cylinder, either circular or rectangular. Figure 5–23 illustrates what happens if a

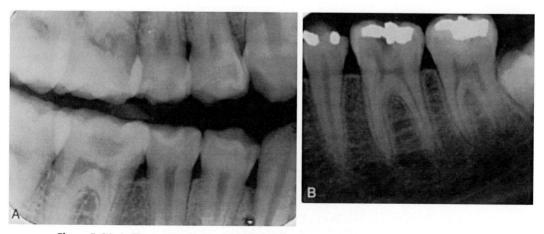

Figure 5–21. *A,* The contacts between all molar teeth are overlapped owing to improper horizontal angulation. *B,* "Open" contacts on a periapical film with correct horizontal angulation.

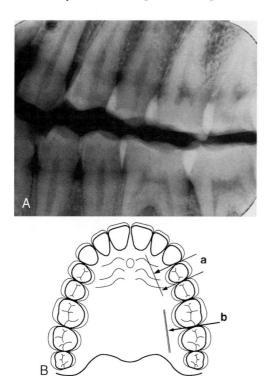

Figure 5–22. *A*, Note here that when the contact area for the distal surfaces of the cuspids is "opened," the contacts posterior to this are "closed," or overlapped. Several views may be required to image all interproximal areas. *B*, The arrows show the different directions from which the central ray (*CR*) must enter to minimize or eliminate overlap; *a* is the premolar view and *b* the molar view.

round cylinder does not cover the film surface correctly. We saw a rectangular cone cut in Figure 5–9. One region where cone cutting commonly occurs is the molar view. The operator is so concerned with "covering" the distal region of the third molar or with showing all the contacts on the bitewing film that he or she moves the tubehead *too far posteriorly*. This results in a cone cut in the bicuspid region. Remember that the interproximal *bitewing* film needs to cover only the contact between the permanent second molar and the wisdom tooth, with no need to extend past the distal surface of the third molar for the molar bitewing view.

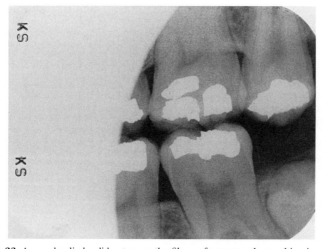

Figure 5–23. A round cylinder did not cover the film surface correctly, resulting in a cone cut.

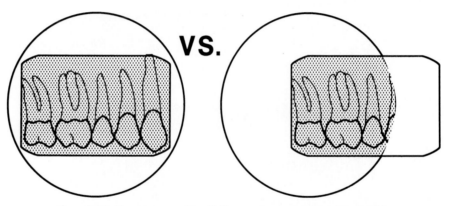

Figure 5–24. Correct cone position (*left*) versus incorrect cone position (*right*).

Figure 5–24 shows both the correct and the incorrect versions of the film placement. This troubleshooting tip will save you frustration (see Fig. 1–24 for further explanation). As for the molar bitewing view, if you ask the patient to part the lips or "grin" (as in Fig. 5–25) and demonstrate with your own lips, you can often see the most anterior edge of the film. The anterior edge of the cylinder should extend slightly beyond this point to ensure total exposure of the area.

Overexposure or Underexposure

Overexposed (dark) films can occur in several ways. One way was discussed in this chapter's "Double Exposure" section. In addition, one can overexpose a film by improper selection of (1) the exposure time (too long) and (2) the kilovoltage peak (kVp). This can also be true for the milliamperage (mA); however, most dental x-ray machines have a fixed milliamperage at either 10 mA or 15 mA.

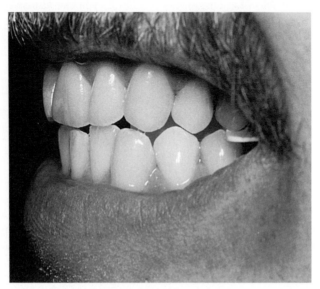

Figure 5–25. Patient parting his lips to allow better visualization of film placement to assist in positioning the cone.

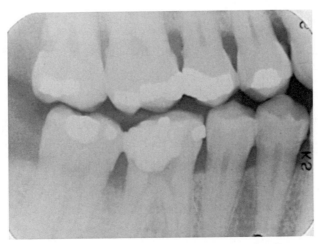

Figure 5–26. This molar film is so underexposed that it is almost impossible to distinguish enamel from dentin. The dentinoenamel junction is not discernible on many teeth. Carious lesions would be impossible to detect.

Many machines also have a kilovoltage peak fixed at 70 kVp or 90 kVp. Therefore, the most common overexposure error is due to improper time selection.

A list of exposure factors in the form of a chart should be posted in all operatories to ensure proper time of exposure. Attention to this chart will help to eliminate overexposure of dental radiographs. But be prepared to use longer times on larger-than-average patients and shorter times on smaller-than-average patients. This rule applies to both adults and children.

Underexposed films can also occur in several ways. If routine exposure factors are selected for the larger-than-average patient, it may be difficult to penetrate the tissues; that is, the thickness of the patient's tissues may not allow the x rays to reach the film. A film placed backward, with the lead foil between the tubehead and the film surface, will also be underexposed (see Figure 5–9).

Just as you can select too long an exposure time, you can also select too short an exposure time. If you have exposed a central incisor region, using Ektaspeed Plus* film six impulses, and you forget to change the exposure time to that appropriate for an Ultra-speed* film (about 10 impulses), the resultant image will be underexposed and undiagnostic. This error may require a retake. Figure 5-26 demonstrates an underexposed image.

Patient Errors

Patient Movement

Just about the only film retake that can be blamed on the patient is that resulting from patient movement. However, the operator *can control or minimize this problem.* Patient movement usually arises from discomfort (owing to improper film placement, failure of the operator to curve the film within reasonable limits, an unsupported patient head position, etc.). These are really operator errors. Patient movement resulting from gagging or swallowing or both can also largely be

---

*Ektaspeed Plus, Ultra-speed, Eastman Kodak Company, Rochester, NY.

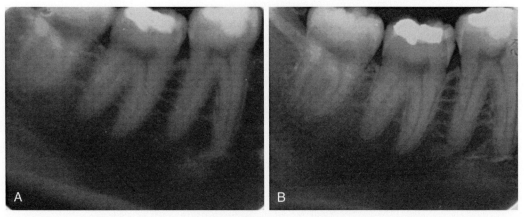

Figure 5–27. Radiographic images with (*A*) and without (*B*) patient movement.

prevented but is sometimes unavoidable. Figure 5–27 demonstrates radiographic images with (*A*) and without (*B*) patient movement.

Film Movement

A film may move in the biteblock because the plastic holder is stretched, owing to wear from bending the backing plate too much or too often (Fig. 5–28*A* and *B*).

A film can also move if the patient moves his or her tongue or swallows. It is sometimes difficult to separate patient and film movement—one is often the result of the other. The results are the same: a blurred image. Some patients will move the head (thus moving the film) in a response to your directions to "sit still" or "don't move" or "close your eyes." The patient often nods agreement. The best result comes from direct observation of the patient at the moment of exposure. If there is movement, do not continue. Reinstruct the patient or reposition the film as necessary.

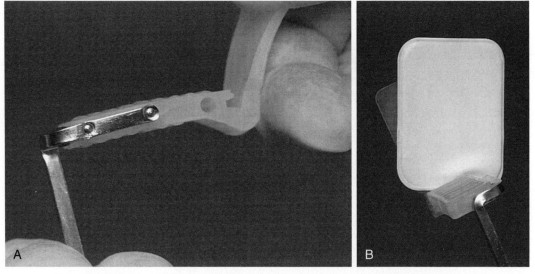

Figure 5–28. Operator bending packing plate. *B,* Film dislodges easily and would be incorrectly positioned in the patient's mouth.

TABLE 5–3. PROCESSING ERRORS

STAINED FILMS	FOGGED FILMS
Fixer artifact	Safelight problems
Developer artifact	Improper film storage
Water stains	**LIGHT FILMS**
Fluoride stains	Development time too short
DARK FILMS	Developer concentration low
Light leaks	Contaminated developer
Development time too long	Excess fixer
Developer concentration high	Temperature too low
Paper stuck to film	
Improper fixation	
Temperature too high	

PROCESSING ERRORS

Successfully exposing the film is only half of the radiographic imaging process. Many films are rendered undiagnostic because of improper film processing. Dental x-ray films, as discussed in Chapter 2, must be processed carefully, with attention to detail, under good safelight conditions, and in a clean environment. Poor chemicals, inadequate development time or temperature, and improper darkroom safelighting are but a few examples of how a quality film can be ruined. Table 5-3 outlines the major processing errors that the operator must avoid.

Stained Films

Any fluid can stain a dental x-ray film. If drops of water on a film are left in contact long enough, they will dissolve the emulsion in the area and leave a clear spot (Fig. 5–29). Some water stains will be dark but translucent because they only dilute the film emulsion and allow it to run (Fig. 5–30). Yellow or brown stains on a radiograph are usually a sign of improper washing or clearing of the *fixer* solution from the film. The excess fixer oxidizes with age and discolors, leaving a yellow or brown stain. Fixer dropped onto an unprocessed film will cause a white spot, usually in a round or ovoid shape (Fig. 5–31).

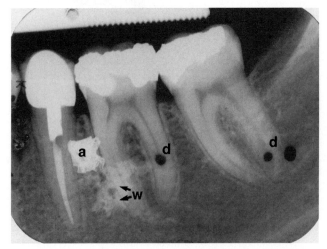

Figure 5–29. Water (*w*) dropped on film; developer spots (*d*) on film; artifact (*a*).

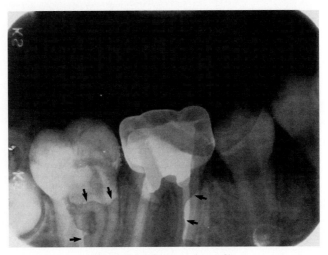

Figure 5–30. Water marks on film.

If developer is dropped or spilled onto a film, the resulting artifact will be dark or black. Other black marks on a radiograph can occur if the film was handled by an operator with *fluoride* on his or her fingers. This artifact appears as a fingerprint (Fig. 5–32).

Fogged Films

We have distinguished fogged films from *dark* films because, although fogged films are dark, they still appear to be relatively normal. Fog may be caused by improper safelighting in the darkroom (light leaks), storage in a warm-to-hot environment, or out-of-date film. The changes in film density as a result of fog are subtle. Fogged films usually appear almost uniformly gray. This uniformity reduces the film's contrast and may obscure dental problems such as early carious lesions in enamel. If there is insufficient contrast (black/white), the gray cavity

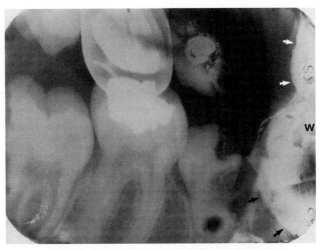

Figure 5–31. This film has multiple processing and handling artifacts. The fixer stain is the white region indicated on the right of the film (*arrows*). Water marks (*w*) are also apparent.

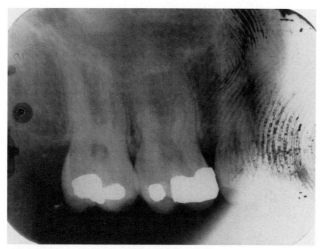

Figure 5–32. Fingerprints are obvious on the right side of the film. The fingers were contaminated with fluoride solution. Can you name two other errors present? Hint: one is a technical error, and the other is a processing error.

may blend into the gray background. Figure 5–33 is an example of a fogged film that is largely uninterpretable because it is so gray.

Dark Films

There are many causes of dark films. We saw in the section on technique errors earlier in this chapter that overexposure leads to an overall dark film, because far more x rays reach the film surface to expose the film. Similarly, light photons (like x-ray photons) striking the film will cause the formation of a latent image center that, when subjected to developer, will turn black. Stray light, then, can expose a dental x-ray film unnecessarily. After all, light is an electromagnetic radiation, just as x rays are.

One of the more common processing errors in which stray light exposes the undeveloped film is caused by loose-fitting fabric openings on the "daylight" hoods or loaders of automatic developers (Fig. 5–34). The quick removal of your hands from these openings could also allow light to expose the film before it has fully entered the developing tank. These errors are easily avoided.

Overdevelopment of a film because of an overly long development time (usually during hand processing) or an overly high (strong) developer concentration (owing to over-replenishment) will result in films that are dark. Additionally, if the fixer concentration is weak, it cannot remove all of the excess developer from the film, and the image will be darker (Fig. 5–35).

Finally, if the operator is in a rush or is not paying proper attention, the wrapping paper from inside the film packet may be placed into the solution along with the film. The paper sticks to the film surface and is developed, fixed, and subsequently "baked" onto the x-ray film in the dryer. This results in an unsalvageable film, a retake, and undue patient exposure. Proper maintenance of processing chemicals and care in film developing (as discussed in Chapter 2) are mandatory to reduce these errors. One positive note is that overexposed or dark films (with the exceptions of chemical stains, light-leak problems, and paper stuck on the

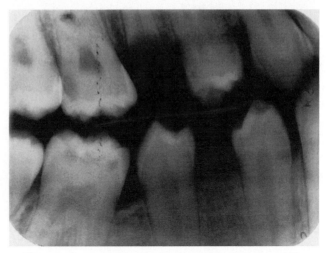

Figure 5–33. An example of a largely uninterpretable, fogged film.

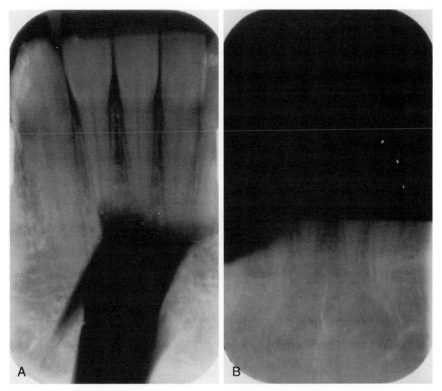

Figure 5–34. *A* and *B*, Black areas on both films were caused by accidental exposure to light. The irregular black artifact in *A* resulted from removing the hands from the daylight loader before the film had fully entered the machine.

Figure 5–35. Overdevelopment. The details, seen here as dots, are not readily discernible. This x ray appears developed correctly in Figure 4–2.

film) can often be viewed under a "hot light" (a bright source) to retrieve some information. Furthermore, duplication of the film using overexposure of the direct positive film may also salvage some information (Figs. 5–36 and 5–37) and thus save the patient additional x-ray exposure.

Light Films

Unfortunately, underexposed, or light, films caused by the following errors are for the most part undiagnostic; that is, they will require a retake. Even if you have properly exposed a film, if your development time is too short or your developer concentration is too weak (exhausted), you may be left with a light film with insufficient contrast or detail for diagnostic interpretation (Fig. 5–38). Other causes of light films are excess fixation, inadequate (too low) developing temperature, and films placed backwards. With the advent of automatic processors, we have an additional cause for light films: the operator may forget to separate the two films

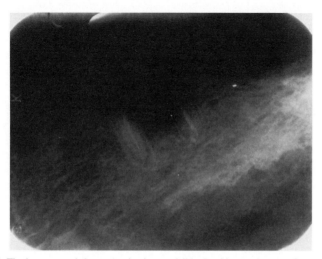

Figure 5–36. The bone around these root tips is not visible. Looking at the manufacturer's film code, only the "K" of the "KS" is visible.

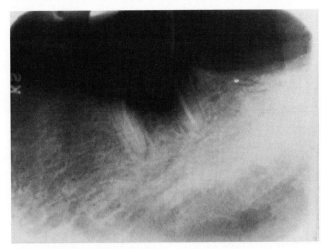

Figure 5–37. Here, more bone is visible as well as both letters of the film code "KS." Even a faint outline of a crown is partially visible.

in a double-film pocket, or one film might be fed into the processor too soon after the other. In both instances, the films stick together either wholly or partially. After they are retrieved, the only solution is to peel them apart and place them back into the *fixer* section for reprocessing prior to exposing them to white light. Even after reprocessing, part or all of the emulsion on one side of the films will not get developed, and the resultant films will be lighter than usual.

A POTPOURRI OF ADDITIONAL ERRORS

- A maxillary complete denture left in the mouth (Fig. 5–39).
- A cast metallic maxillary partial denture left in the mouth (Fig. 5–40).
- An acrylic orthodontic appliance left in the mouth, of which only the retentive clasp can be seen (Fig. 5–41).
- Chewing gum left in the mouth (Fig. 5–42).
- A finger superimposed over the mouth (Fig. 5–43).
- A "fingernail" artifact (Fig. 5–44).

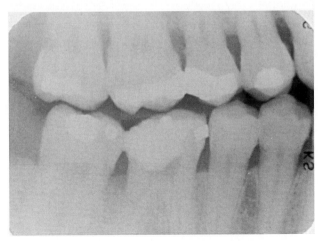

Figure 5–38. A light film owing to short development time or weak developer concentration.

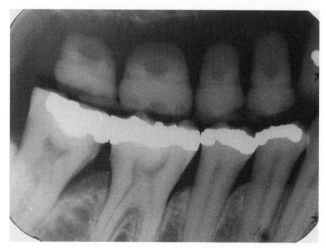

Figure 5–39. It is sometimes beneficial to leave the prosthesis in the patient's mouth to assist with correct placement. Here the bitewing radiograph is stabilized by the denture; without it, the film would probably have tipped.

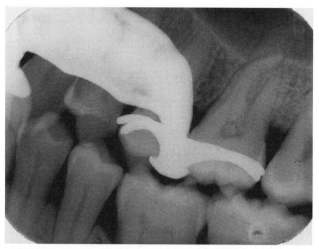

Figure 5–40. In this case the metallic framework of the partial denture obscures interproximal contact areas and bony detail.

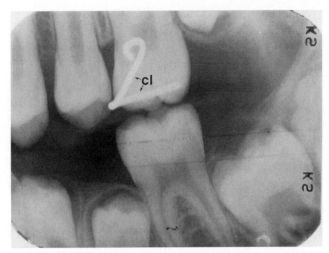

Figure 5–41. Because the partial denture is made of acrylic (plastic), it is not visible on the film. Only the wrought wire clasp (*cl*) used for retention on this side is visible.

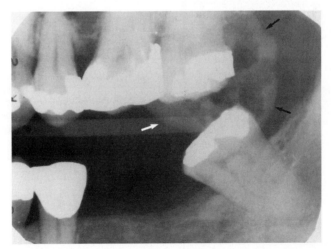

Figure 5–42. Chewing gum (*arrows*). Note the indentations (bitemarks) present.

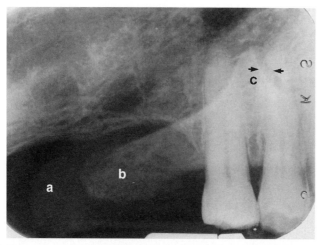

Figure 5–43. This patient was holding a film in the mouth during a bisecting angle procedure. The index finger was behind the film on the palate, and the thumb was outside the arch between the film and the source. Thus, *a* is the soft tissue of the end of the finger, *b* is the distal phalanx and terminal tuft, and *c* is the distal interphalangeal joint. This artifact has been facetiously called a "phalangioma" by some authors.

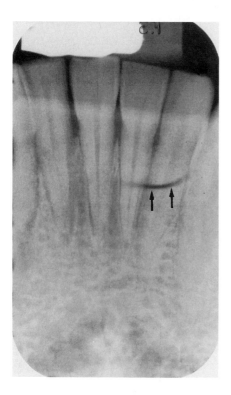

Figure 5–44. If the operator has difficulty removing the film from the packet, he or she may grasp the film between the fingernails of two fingers and cause a crease or crimping artifact. This is termed by some a "fingernail artifact" (*arrow*).

Study Questions

1. You develop a set of bitewings in an automatic processer; three are good, but one is totally blank, with no hint of an image. What can you assume about the blank film?
   A. It was exposed to light.
   B. It was put in the fixer solution first.
   C. It was not exposed to radiation.
   D. It was double-exposed.
2. You look at the bitewings you took during Mrs. Jones's last appointment 1 year ago. They are brownish and somewhat opaque, not very usable. You look at her chart and see a note that said she was 20 minutes late for her last appointment, which was the last appointment of the day. Then you remember how you hurried to get the films processed and hung up to dry so you could go home. What might be the cause of the film discoloration?
   A. The films were not developed long enough.
   B. The films were not fixed or washed long enough.
   C. The films were exposed to light leaks in the darkroom.
   D. The films were developed too long.
3. You turn on the water in the manual tanks at the beginning of the day, stir the solution, check the temperature, and set a developing time to go with the temperature. You take a set of films at about 9 a.m. that appear fine. About 2 p.m., you process another set of films that are so dark you can hardly read them. What most likely happened with the second set of films?
   A. Your exposure time was too long.
   B. Your darkroom has a light leak.
   C. Your water temperature is too hot.
   D. Your chemicals are contaminated.
4. You take a set of bitewings, and they all have a few little black spots on them. The most likely cause is
   A. Developer splashed on them.
   B. Fixer splashed on them.
   C. Water splashed on them.
   D. All of the above.
5. You notice that over the last few weeks the films have been getting lighter and lighter. No difference is noticeable from one day to the next, but there is a big difference between a periapical you did on Mr. Smith today and his bitewings from 2 weeks ago. What could be the cause of the films getting lighter?
   A. Light leaks.
   B. Weak or contaminated developer.
   C. Weak or contaminated fixer.
   D. Overly short exposure time.

6. You finish taking films and start to dismiss the patient as you clean up the bracket tray with scalers and fluoride trays on it. Then you realize that the patient was supposed to have bitewings taken. You quickly do the bitewings and process them. You pick up your processed films from the automatic processor and notice that there are fingerprints on them. What could have caused the fingerprints?

   A. The emulsion began to soften before you got the films into the processor.

   B. There may be some kind of light leak in the darkroom that caused the image of your fingers to show up on the films.

   C. Your fingers may have had fluoride on them, which caused the artifacts.

   D. None of the above.

7. You are preparing to mount the complete mouth radiographic series (CMRS) that you have laid out on the viewbox in front of you. You notice that one film is blank. The other films look normal except for one that seems somewhat darker than the others. What most likely caused the blank and dark films?

   A. The x-ray unit malfunctioned.

   B. The films were incorrectly processed.

   C. The film-holding device was assembled incorrectly.

   D. The clear film was placed in the fixer first.

   E. One film was double-exposed, and one was unexposed.

Chapter 6

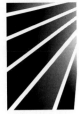

Accessory Radiographic Techniques and Patient Management

BISECTING-ANGLE TECHNIQUE

The bisecting-angle technique is based on a geometric principle of equally dividing a triangle. This technique differs from the paralleling technique in that, instead of moving the film away from the teeth to make the film and teeth parallel, the operator places the film directly against the teeth to be radiographed (Fig. 6–1).

You will notice in Figure 6–1 that the film touches the teeth at the incisal edge, or lingual-occlusal surface. The apical portion of the film is held away from the teeth at a distance determined by the patient's anatomy. Thus, the film is not parallel to the teeth but meets the teeth at an angle.

If we direct the x-ray beam at a right angle to the film, the image produced on the film will be much shorter than the actual structure: the image will be foreshortened (see Fig. 5–18). If we direct the x-ray beam perpendicular to the long axes of the teeth, the image produced on the film will be much longer than the actual structure: the image will be elongated (see Fig. 5–19). The bisecting-angle technique combines these positions to obtain a reasonably accurate image.

With this technique, the angle formed by the long axes of the teeth and the film is bisected into two equal parts, and the x-ray beam is directed perpendicular to the bisecting line (Fig. 6–1). This concept is simple to explain, but the technique is rather difficult to employ so that a quality radiograph is obtained. Problems are posed by the fact that (1) the operator cannot see the long axes of the teeth and therefore must estimate their correct orientation; (2) the operator must *imagine* the line that bisects the angle that cannot be seen; (3) the operator cannot see exactly where the film is and thus cannot be sure that the cylinder will cover the entire area of the film; and (4) the patient, in many instances, must hold the film in place

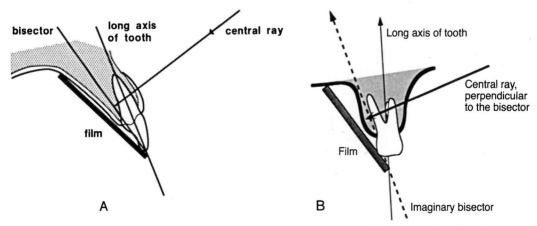

Figure 6–1. A, A diagram of an anterior tooth with the central ray perpendicular to the "imaginary" bisector of the angle between the long axis of the tooth and the film plane. *B*, A posterior tooth using the bisecting-angle concept.

with a finger, which may result in film bending or in improper film positioning. Consequently, this technique may result in more operator and patient errors than the paralleling technique, which uses positioning devices.

Exposure Factors

The bisecting-angle technique uses a short source-to-film distance (SFD) of 7 or 8 inches (cylinder length). This shorter distance allows reduced exposure times (recall the inverse square law stated in Chapter 4) of approximately one-fourth those used in the paralleling technique, with a 14- or 16-inch SFD. The shorter distance, however, has two negative effects on the film and on the patient: (1) the shorter distance creates greater magnification of the entire image on the film (Fig. 6–2), and (2) the shorter SFD of the bisecting-angle technique causes the x-ray beam to cover a greater area of the head, thus adding to the patient's absorbed dose (see Figs. 3–14 and 4–8).

Film Placement

The number of films used and their *placement* (anterior/posterior positions) in the bisecting-angle technique are similar to the number and placement of films in the paralleling technique. The *horizontal angle* is determined similarly, except that the metal arm of the positioning instrument is not present as a visual guide. *Vertical placement* of the film should allow 1/8 to 1/4 inch of the film packet to extend above the occlusal line on mandibular films and below the occlusal line on maxillary films. The *vertical angle* is determined by the bisector line, as described previously.

Uses

Because of the increased potential for operator and patient error, greater image distortion, and increased radiation dose to the patient, the bisecting-angle technique is not recommended as a standard technique by the authors. The bisecting-angle technique does have use in dental radiography in some circumstances, such as with difficult or unusual patient anatomy, disabling conditions that prevent the patient from biting on a biteblock, uncooperative patients such as small children,

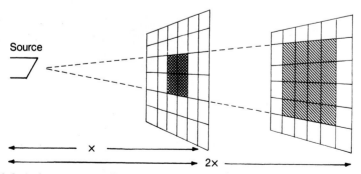

Figure 6–2. A shorter source-to-film distance creates greater magnification of the entire image on the film.

and some endodontic films. The operator should be aware of both the usefulness *and* the limitations of this technique.

OCCLUSAL RADIOGRAPHY

A supplementary technique to periapical and bitewing radiography is occlusal radiography. This technique uses a larger film that can be placed in the mouth as if the patient were biting a sandwich (Fig. 6–3).

Uses and Advantages

Occlusal radiography can be used in the following situations:

1. To determine the location of objects in all three dimensions.
2. To locate roots as well as supernumerary, unerupted, and impacted teeth (i.e., canines, third molars).

Film Placement. Long or short dimension of the film across the mouth.

Vertical Angulation. (+) 70 to 75 degrees downward.

Point of Entry of Central Ray. At the bridge of the nose.

Pediatric Patient. Use the size no. 2 (periapical) film, because small children may not be able to accommodate the larger occlusal film in their mouths.

Approximate Exposure. 90 kVp, 10 mA. Adult: 12 to 15 impulses. Child: 8 to 10 impulses.

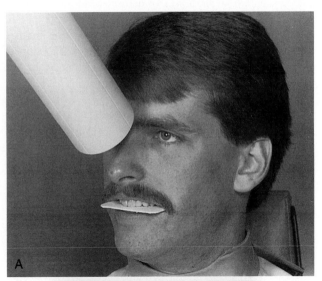

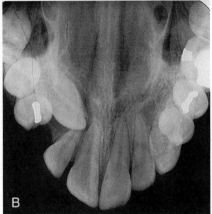

Figure 6–3. A, The patient positioned for a topographic maxillary occlusal view. *B,* The topographic maxillary occlusal view affords an excellent view of the palate.

3. To localize foreign bodies in the jaws and stones in the salivary gland ducts.
4. To visualize and evaluate the integrity of the anterior, medial, and lateral outlines of the maxillary sinus.
5. To determine the nature, extent, and displacement of fractures of the mandible and maxilla.
6. To determine the presence and extent of pathoses, such as cysts, osteomyelitis, and malignancies.
7. To demonstrate bony expansion of either the maxilla or the mandible.
8. To examine larger segments of the jaw (maxilla and mandible) (by virtue of the larger film size used).
9. For patients who are unable to open the mouth wide enough for periapical radiographs because of trismus, pain, or other reasons.
10. For pediatric patients when intraoral periapical films are difficult to obtain.

With pediatric patients, occlusal films can be used for localization of objects, that is, to help determine whether an object is positioned facially or lingually to the arches. Occlusal radiographs are also often used to examine the arches for symmetry or cortical bone expansion.

Two standard angulations can be used with the occlusal radiographic technique, each giving a slightly different view. The first is the topographic view, a technique that is somewhat similar to the bisecting-angle technique. The dental arch to be radiographed is positioned parallel to the floor. The film is placed in the patient's mouth. The central ray is directed perpendicular to the line that bisects the angle

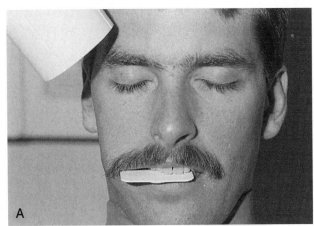
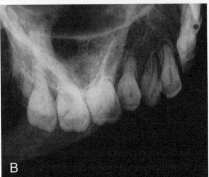

Head Position. Occlusal plane horizontal.

Film Position. Sensitive side up. Film positioned in the mouth with one of the long edges of the packet lying parallel to, and extending 1/4 inch (6 to 7 mm) beyond, the buccal cusps of the posterior teeth. Teeth closed gently on the film packet.

Vertical Angulation. (+) 60 degrees downward.

Horizontal Angulation. Depending on the view required, beam angulation may be at a right angle to the buccal plane of the cuspid or at a right angle to the buccal plane of the molar or bicuspid teeth, similar to the bisecting angle technique.

Approximate Exposure. 90 kVp, 10 mA. Adult: 12 to 15 impulses. Child: 8 to 10 impulses.

Figure 6–4. A and *B,* Occlusal film placed to one side of the arch (*right*) for examination of that side.

formed by the long axis of the anterior teeth and the plane of the film. The topographic view gives a reasonably accurate image of the anterior teeth, although the posterior teeth are superimposed over themselves. This technique gives essentially an enlarged periapical view (Figs. 6–3 through 6–5).

The second standard angulation is the *cross-sectional technique,* in which the film is placed between the teeth and the central ray and angled 90 degrees perpendicular to the film. *Impulse times are given for use with Ektaspeed film* (Fig. 6–6).

Topographic Maxillary Occlusal View. This film affords an excellent view of the palate.

Maxillary Lateral (Right/Left) Occlusal View. This view depicts palatal roots of molar teeth. It may be used to locate foreign bodies in the antrum or to demonstrate larger lesions of the maxilla.

Topographic Mandibular Occlusal View. This view should show the inferior border of the anterior mandible in its entirety. Use a size no. 2 film for a small child.

Cross-Sectional Mandibular Occlusal View. This film affords views of the buccal and lingual aspects of the mandible as well as the location of sialoliths and foreign bodies in the floor of the mouth.

As with the maxillary view, the mandibular occlusal film can be positioned over the right or left side of the mandibular arch only. Figure 6–7 illustrates how the position of the film varies for this technique. The angles and exposure factors are the same as for the standard *cross-sectional mandibular occlusal view.* The expo-

Head Position. Tilted back to a comfortable position. Median sagittal plane vertical.

Film Position. Sensitive side facing mandibular teeth. Long dimension across the mouth. Teeth closed gently on the film packet.

Vertical Angulation. Determined by bisecting principles.

Point of Entry of Central Ray (CR). Just below the apices of the mandibular teeth, or about 1/4 inch (6 to 7 mm) above the tip of the chin (along its median line).

Horizontal Angulation. CR follows the median sagittal line.

Approximate Exposure. 90 kVp, 10 mA. Adult: 12 to 15 impulses. Child: 8 to 10 impulses.

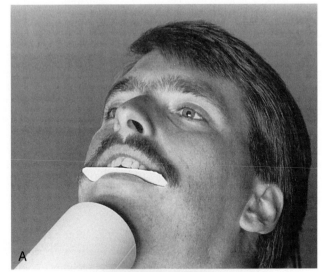

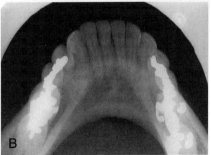

Figure 6–5. A and *B,* Topographic mandibular occlusal view.

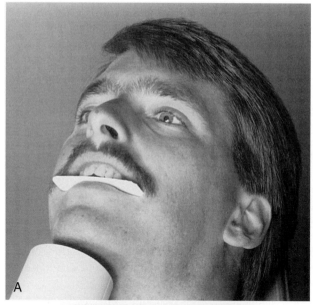

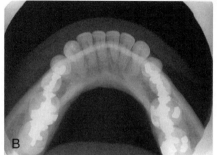

Head Position. Tilted as far back as comfort will allow. The median sagittal plane is vertical.

Film Position. Sensitive side facing the mandibular teeth. Short/long dimension across the mouth, depending on the width/length of the arch.

Vertical Angulation. Direct CR perpendicular to the plane of the film.

Point of Entry of Central Ray. Opposite the first molar along the median line under the chin. Move the beam about 2 inches (5 cm) from the underside of the chin to minimize cone cutting.

Horizontal Angulation. CR follows the median plane.

Approximate Exposure. 90 kVp, 10 mA. Adult: 12 to 15 impulses. Child: 8 to 10 impulses.

Figure 6–6. A and B, Cross-sectional technique (view).

sure times are approximate and may vary based on inherent differences in machines and the length of the cone.

PEDIATRIC RADIOGRAPHIC TECHNIQUE

Management of the behavior of the pediatric patient is the key to successful technique. With children, you have to be imaginative, creative, entertaining, quick-witted, and patient. Here are some basic guidelines to consider when your patient is a child:

1. **Show children what you are going to do** every chance you get. Talk about the "pictures" you are going to take and the "camera" you are going to use. Let them touch the equipment, push the exposure button (while the unit is off, of course), touch the film, and see what a radiograph looks like. You might even bring an extra film packet and positioning instrument to place into your own mouth for demonstration. Show them that you are comfortable with it in place.

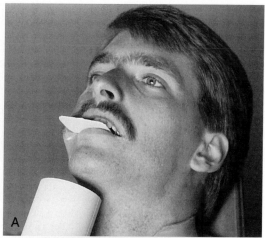

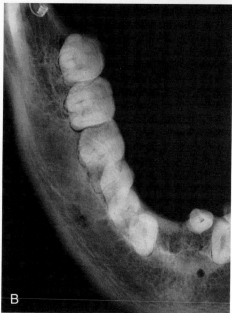

Figure 6–7. A and B, A variation in the positioning of the mandibular occlusal film.

2. **Work quickly.** Remember that many children move continually. Tell them the importance of staying perfectly still. Reinforce any positive behavior with praise.
3. **Be creative.** If your regular technique does not work, improvise. Be prepared to substitute smaller films or occlusal films, etc.

Technique

Protection. Because children are growing and developing, their tissues are generally at higher risk for radiation-induced problems. It is imperative to follow good patient radiation protection procedures. Use of a leaded apron and a thyroid shield is critical with children.

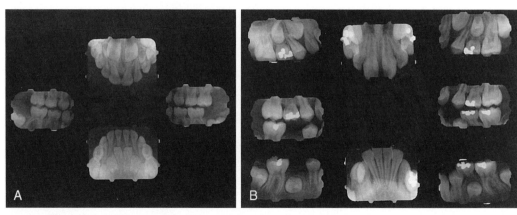

Figure 6–8. A, This survey would be used for a 3- to 5-year-old patient. It employs two size no. 1 films for bitewing and radiographs and two size no. 2 films for maxillary and mandibular occlusal views. *B,* This survey would be used for a child with a mixed dentition (age 6–10 years). It uses four size no. 1 films as periapicals in addition to the films listed for part *A.*

Type of Radiographic Survey. The need for a complete mouth radiographic survey (CMRS) for children is variable. Selection of the number, size, and type of film depends on the child's age and size as well as the amount of patient cooperation given. Figure 6–8 shows examples of some pediatric surveys using different types of films.

Alterations in Exposure Factors. Exposure factors are generally reduced for children. Less exposure time and sometimes less milliamperage can be employed. Because children's tissues are often not as thick as adults', they require less radiation. It is best to decrease the exposure time rather than the milliamperage, because children often move. A shorter exposure time reduces the probability of a motion artifact (blurring). The exact exposure settings depend on the size of the child. Furthermore, if the child is very small, a booster seat may be necessary for proper beam alignment.

Film Size. Use the smallest film size that is compatible with the patient's anatomy. The use of oversized film will cause discomfort and loss of cooperation. For a primary dentition, size no. 0 film is recommended. Size no. 0 or size no. 1 may be used for a child with mixed dentition. Sizes no. 1 and 2 may be used for preadolescent and adolescent dentitions.

Bitewings. Normally, until the second molars have erupted, only two bitewings are necessary, as all erupted posterior teeth will usually fit on one film.

EDENTULOUS RADIOGRAPHIC TECHNIQUE

Radiographs of edentulous patients are some of the most difficult to perform. Because the incidence of pathology can be high in edentulous areas, a CMRS may be indicated. Also, prior to denture construction it may be necessary to determine the proximity of the mandibular canals or maxillary sinuses to the alveolar ridge crest. Some dentists or dental specialists who perform implants may use these films to assess bone height and bone quality, as well as to visualize anatomic structures such as the sinus floor or mental foramen.

Films

A typical survey may contain as many as 14 (six anterior and eight posterior) or as few as 10 (two anterior and eight posterior) periapical films (Fig. 6–9). Bitewings are not taken because there are no teeth.

Technique

Either the bisecting-angle or the paralleling technique may be used for edentulous radiographs. Because there are no teeth, the distortion inherent in the bisecting-angle technique does not interfere with diagnosis of intrabony conditions; remember, however, that the patient receives more radiation from this technique.

If the bisecting-angle technique is chosen, films should be placed so that 1/4 inch of the film is above or below the alveolar ridge. If the paralleling technique is used with instruments, cotton roll(s) may be attached to the biteblock with rubber bands for support (Fig. 6–10). Paralleling techniques also give more accurate views for assessment of bone height before implant surgery.

Exposure Factors

The exposure time for each region should be reduced by approximately one-fourth the normal time to avoid overexposure (and thus dark films), because the bone may be thinner and because there are no teeth.

Alternative Film Surveys

Occlusal films with posterior periapicals or a correctly positioned and exposed panoramic film may be acceptable alternatives for a CMRS with the edentulous patient.

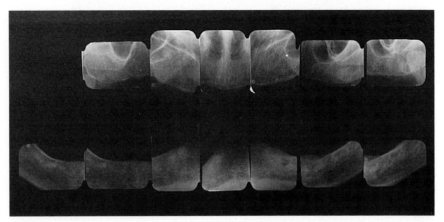

Figure 6–9. This series of 13 films was taken prior to construction of complete upper and lower dentures.

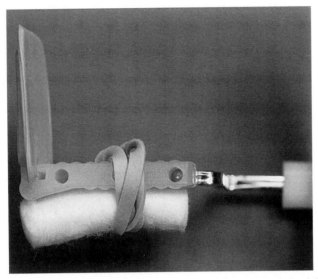

Figure 6–10. A biteblock with a single cotton roll attached to it with an elastic band. More than one cotton roll may have to be attached. Usually the cotton rolls are placed on the block opposite the ridge to be photographed.

ENDODONTIC RADIOGRAPHIC TECHNIQUE

Accurate films are essential for diagnosis, treatment, and follow-up care in endodontic patients. Endodontic films are difficult to obtain during treatment because of rubber dam clamps, instruments, or obturating material extending from the tooth (Fig. 6–11). Aside from these physical problems, visualization of correct film placement is difficult because the rubber dam obstructs the view. A diagnostic endodontic film should ensure that (1) the tooth is centered on the film; (2) at least

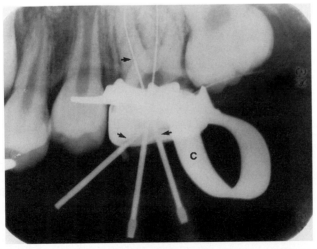

Figure 6–11. This radiograph demonstrates an attempt to image the apices of the maxillary left first permanent molar. The rubber dam clamp *(c)* and gutta-percha points *(arrows)* make film placement difficult. The apex of the molar is not visible; to include it would require a retake.

5 mm of bone beyond the apex of the tooth is visible; and (3) the image is as anatomically correct as possible.

The preoperative diagnostic film and the postoperative follow-up film should be taken using the standard paralleling technique. *The bisecting-angle* technique is not recommended because of the inherent dimensional distortion.

Anterior Films

Films may be held parallel to the long axis of the tooth by means of a hemostat, a Snap-a-Ray,* a tongue depressor, or a finger (Fig. 6–12). If this approach cannot be used, cotton rolls may be taped to the film to hold it away from the tooth to maintain the most parallel relationship possible (Fig. 6–13). If neither of these methods will work, the bisecting-angle technique can be used as long as the clinician is aware of the dimensional and linear distortion that will result.

Posterior Films

The paralleling technique is superior to the bisecting-angle technique for posterior films as well as anterior films. If films can be held parallel to the long axis of the tooth by use of a hemostat or a Snap-a-Ray, the accuracy of the film will be maximized (Fig. 6–14). If this approach is not possible, a cotton roll may be taped to the film to hold it farther from the tooth, making it more parallel to the tooth.

---

*Dentsply Rinn Corporation; Elgin, IL.

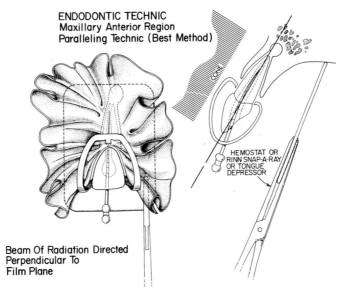

ENDODONTIC TECHNIC
Maxillary Anterior Region
Paralleling Technic (Best Method)

HEMOSTAT OR
RINN SNAP-A-RAY
OR TONGUE
DEPRESSOR

Beam Of Radiation Directed
Perpendicular To
Film Plane

Figure 6–12. Film held parallel to the long axis of an endodontically treated tooth. (Courtesy of Dr. John Preece, University of Texas Health Science Center, San Antonio, TX.)

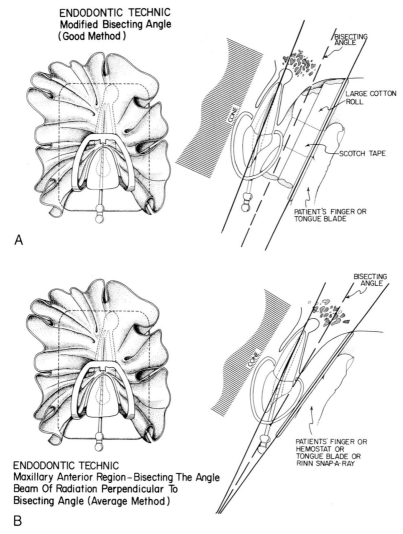

ENDODONTIC TECHNIC
Modified Bisecting Angle
(Good Method)

BISECTING
ANGLE

LARGE COTTON
ROLL

SCOTCH TAPE

PATIENT'S FINGER OR
TONGUE BLADE

A

BISECTING
ANGLE

ENDODONTIC TECHNIC
Maxillary Anterior Region – Bisecting The Angle
Beam Of Radiation Perpendicular To
Bisecting Angle (Average Method)

PATIENTS' FINGER OR
HEMOSTAT OR
TONGUE BLADE OR
RINN SNAP-A-RAY

B

Figure 6–13. *A,* An alternative technique using a tongue blade and cotton rolls. *B,* A bisecting alternative. This technique involves more distortion. (Courtesy of Dr. John Preece, University of Texas Health Science Center, San Antonio, TX.)

LOCALIZATION TECHNIQUES

Right-angle Technique

Sometimes the operator needs to know if an object—for example, an impacted tooth—is located toward the buccal (facial) or lingual portion of the mandibular arch. The right-angle technique (also called Miller's technique) is a simple method for determining the facial/lingual position of teeth or foreign objects.

Method

Two radiographs are taken at right angles to each other. The first radiograph may be a periapical or bitewing already available from a survey. This film will

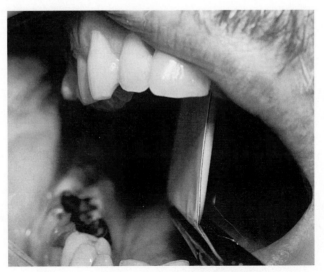

Figure 6–14. Film held in the mouth in a parallel position.

show the position of the object in an *inferior/superior and anterior/posterior* direction. The second film is a cross-sectional occlusal projection, using an occlusal- or periapical-size film. This film will show the *facial/lingual* and *anterior/posterior* position. Using the differing views given by the two films, you can pinpoint the object in three dimensions. This technique is used primarily for locating objects in the mandibular arch (Fig. 6–15).

BUCCAL OBJECT RULE

The *buccal object rule* (also known as Clark's rule and the "Same on Lingual, Opposite on Buccal"—SLOB—rule) can be used if two films are already available with slightly different angles or positions. The principle of the buccal object rule states that the object closest to the buccal surface will appear to move in the opposite direction relative to the movement of the tubehead when a second film is taken (Fig. 6–16). An additional illustration of this rule and an explanation of the SLOB rule are found in Chapter 12, Figure 12–39.

Method

If you have two objects directly in line with each other and you stand in line with them, the object farthest away will be blocked from your view. But if you (not the objects) move to the side, it *appears* that the object closest to you moves in the opposite direction.

Near objects (which would be buccal) appear to move in the *opposite* direction relative to the direction that the tube moved. Far objects (which would be lingual) appear to move in the *same* direction that the tube moved.

It may be helpful to remember the name "*b*uccal *o*bject rule" and the fact that *b*uccal objects appear to move in the *o*pposite direction of the tube.

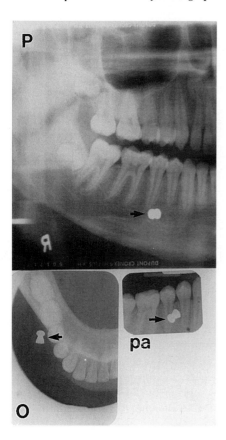

Figure 6–15. The initial radiographs taken were the panoramic (*P*) and the periapical (*pa*) views. These views give the impression that the radiopaque object (a pellet, labeled by arrows) is the bone. A third film, an occlusal view (*O*), reveals that the pellet is really in soft tissue on the outside, or buccal to the mandible.

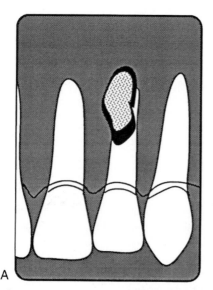
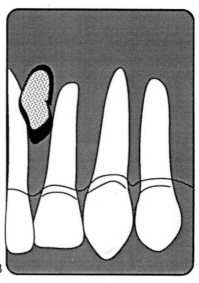

Figure 6–16. As the operator shifted the tubehead posteriorly to move from a lateral incisor view (*A*) to a cuspid view (*B*), the object above the apices moved anteriorly (opposite to the tube shift). Therefore, the object is on the buccal aspect, applying the buccal object rule.

PATIENT MANAGEMENT

Many patients consider radiographic procedures to be unpleasant, especially if the patients have had previous negative experiences. Without patient cooperation the radiographer is greatly handicapped in the attempt to produce quality films. Additionally, patients often transfer their previous negative feelings about the procedure to the current operator. This section of the chapter suggests ways to make the experience more acceptable to the patient and less stressful for the operator.

Operator Attitude

In your initial attempts at radiography, you may be unsure of yourself. Patients are often aware of this, and you may feel your confidence undermined, especially when the patient questions the procedure.

The first requisite for your success and for a less stressful experience is to maintain an air of confidence and authority, *whether you feel it or not.* Remember, if you were not capable of exposing films successfully on a patient, your instructor would not let you begin. Have faith that you have the proper skills and be confident. You should also be familiar with potential problems and how to deal with them.

Just as important as confidence is the knowledge that, between you and the patient, you are the expert. If film placement is uncomfortable, the patient may try to dictate what you should do. If so, remember that you have been taught how to produce quality films, and the patient usually has not. You, therefore, are the one who should control the situation. Following are some useful tips to increase your success:

1. *Try to relax the patient.* Chat with the patient. Explain what you are about to do. Be prepared to answer questions about the hazards of radiation such as how much exposure will be received and the necessity for the films.
2. *Be as gentle as possible, and place films quickly and precisely.* Describe as clearly as possible what you want the patient to do and let him or her know when it is being done correctly. Praise and encouragement will help make patients cooperative. If the patient is not following instructions correctly, keep working with him or her until film placement is correct.

Gagging

One of the more common problems is the patient who gags. Gagging is a physiologic reaction greatly influenced by psychological factors. If you can overcome the psychological barriers, you will increase your chances for a successful experience. The following tips may be useful.

1. *Do not discuss gagging with the patient in advance.* This discussion would just reinforce any thoughts about gagging that the patient may be having.
2. *Start with films that do not normally trigger the gag reflex*—For example, the maxillary central incisor projection. If you start with anterior films and are successful, you will show the patient *that you have the ability and skill*

to place films and that he or she can tolerate them. If the patient gags with later views, he or she must assume some of the responsibility. You have already demonstrated that you can do your part of the procedure.

3. *Do as much as you can in preparation for the exposure before placing a film in the patient's mouth.* Turn the unit on, select the exposure factors, and position the tubehead and the chair as close to the final position as possible before you place the film in the patient's mouth. Use quick, precise movements to place the film. If you try to coax the film into the mouth slowly, you may trigger the gag reflex before the patient begins to close on the biteblock.

4. *Have the patient begin to take deep breaths before you place the film.* Then have him or her breathe **through the mouth** while you are placing the film. Tell the patient that this should keep him or her from gagging. This gives the patient something to concentrate on besides gagging and reinforces the thought that he or she will not gag.

5. *If the patient gags anyway, do not panic.* Simply remove the film and try something else. Distraction techniques work well.

6. You may choose to anesthetize the mouth area. Some mouthwashes or throat lozenges contain a mild anesthetic. These work best if the patient is made to believe they will stop the gag reflex. (Remember, the psychological factor has a big influence.) A topical anesthetic should be considered only in extreme cases, after all other techniques have failed. There are some drawbacks to using topical anesthetics. For example, care should be taken when using an anesthetic in the form of a fine spray, because it might be inhaled into the patient's lungs, causing a toxic reaction.

7. In a few people the gag reflex is so severe that intraoral films are not possible. If none of the techniques described above work, you may consider alternative projections such as panoramic, lateral jaw, or other extraoral films.

PATIENTS WITH DISABILITIES

The problems associated with disabled patients vary with the disability and with its degree of severity. A problem frequently encountered with wheelchair patients is getting them close enough to the x-ray unit. If the patient chooses to or must remain in the wheelchair, the arm of the x-ray unit may be able to be extended to accommodate radiographic procedures. You should be prepared for this necessity in advance. X-ray operatories may have to be rearranged to make the necessary accommodations.

A patient who experiences spastic movements may also make radiography difficult. The patient may be unable to hold films or to bite properly on biteblocks. In such cases, the parent, guardian, or aide accompanying the patient can be asked to hold the films during the procedure. This person should wear a lead apron, thyroid shield, and, if possible, leaded gloves for radiation protection. Extraoral films may be indicated for patients who have uncontrolled movements.

ANATOMIC CONSIDERATIONS

Maxillary Tori

Patients may present a variety of anatomic variations that require a compromise of normal radiographic technique. A maxillary torus is not difficult to work around.

The largest part of the bony structure is directly in the center of the palate, where the vault is the highest and the film packet is usually placed. The torus may prevent film placement high enough in the palate to capture the image of the molar apices. In this situation, the film packet is placed on the opposite side of the torus from the teeth to be radiographed. The added distance from the film to the teeth being radiographed might cause the film to lie at a slightly greater angle to the teeth. This angle could result in foreshortening, although the apices will be imaged with little loss of quality. The shadow of the torus will be superimposed over the apices but will be recognizable. *Care must be used to avoid scraping the sensitive mucosa covering the torus.*

Mandibular Tori

Mandibular tori may be more difficult than maxillary tori to work around. The space between the teeth and the tongue is smaller than that of the palatal vault. You should move the film away from the torus and toward the tongue. If you place your finger between the torus and the film packet, you can then slide the film into place without scraping the overlying mucosa.

Ankyloglossia: The "Tongue-Tied" Patient

When the lingual frenum is attached high on the lingual surface of the mandible or close to the tip of the tongue, the patient has restricted movement, and there is little room to place the film. In this instance, the film can be placed on top of the patient's tongue (Fig. 6–17). The film will still be held in place by the patient closing on the biteblock; the vertical angle may not be quite parallel, but this is acceptable under the circumstances. The soft-tissue shadow of the tongue will be present on the film but should not interfere greatly with its diagnostic quality.

Narrow Palatal Vault

When the arch is extremely narrow, some slight change in normal technique may help. The most important factor is to be sure that *narrow film (size no. 1) is used* for anterior projections. You may have to radiograph each tooth individually in order to obtain quality films without excessive overlap or film bending. Film bending is the most common error associated with this condition. Some people recommend curling the film in order to get it into the narrow arch (Fig. 6–18). Curling will distort the entire image, reduce the diagnostic quality, and possibly lead to a retake; the authors do not recommend it.

Misaligned Teeth

When the patient's teeth are misaligned, you must use your judgment to determine the correct horizontal angulation. Most often, misaligned teeth dictate the need for an extra film. The rotated or malpositioned tooth must be radiographed separately in order to obtain open contacts or a clear view of the roots.

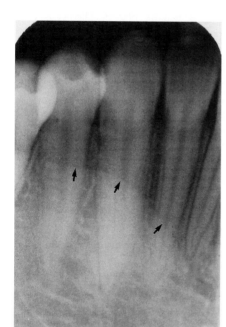

Figure 6–17. Soft-tissue shadow of tongue (*arrows*). Note that its superimposition makes the root more radiopaque (i.e., whiter). The film, however, is still diagnostic.

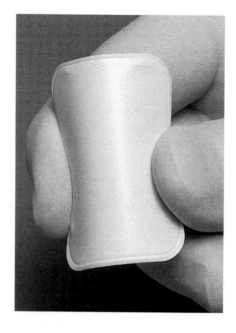

Figure 6–18. The authors do *not* recommend curling the film.

Study Questions

1. Which of the following patients would be most likely to require a 20-film CMRS with 16 periapicals and four bitewings?
   A. A 4-year-old child.
   B. An 8-year-old child.
   C. A 25-year-old edentulous patient.
   D. A 68-year-old dentulous patient.

2. In the bisecting-angle technique, the vertical angle of the central ray is directed
   A. Parallel to the long axis of the tooth.
   B. Parallel to the film.
   C. Perpendicular to the long axis of the tooth.
   D. Perpendicular to a line bisecting the angle made by the long axis of the tooth and the film.
   E. Parallel to a line bisecting the angle made by the long axis of the tooth and the film.

3. As you view a CMRS to record radiographic findings, you notice a well-defined radiopaque object on the film that is obviously not part of the tooth. The object is superimposed over the mesial root of the mandibular first molar in the molar film. As you look at the premolar film, you notice that the object appears to have moved distally and is now closer to the distal root of the first molar. Which of the following statements is true?
   A. The object is in a lingual position.
   B. The object is in a facial position.
   C. You cannot tell from these films where the object is located.
   D. As you moved the film packets forward, you probably pushed the object backward.

4. In order to localize the posterior/anterior position of a broken instrument tip in the mandibular premolar area, you would take a standard periapical film. To localize the precise facial/lingual position for removal, which of the following films would be the best choice?
   A. Cross-sectional occlusal.
   B. Topographical occlusal.
   C. Bitewing.
   D. None of these will localize the facial/lingual position, only the posterior/anterior position.

5. You have to take a periapical film of the right maxillary canine using the bisecting-angle technique. The film has extremely long but well-defined images of the teeth with the apices cut off. What technique error might you suspect?
   A. Horizontal angulation that is too steep.
   B. The patient moved the film while you were not looking.
   C. Vertical angulation that is too steep.
   D. Horizontal angulation that is not steep enough.
   E. Vertical angulation that is not steep enough.

6. A mandibular cross-sectional occlusal film requires
   A. An x-ray beam perpendicular to the film.
   B. A vertical angle of 70 to 75 degrees.
   C. A large film-holding device.
   D. A no. 3 size film.

7. If a patient is suspected of having a bone lesion, such as a cyst, in the posterior area of the mandible, which of the following films would give the best indication of the facial or lingual bony expansion?
   A. A molar periapical using the bisecting-angle technique.
   B. A mandibular occlusal film.
   C. An endodontic film using a hemostat or tongue blade to hold the film in place.
   D. A no. 3 or no. 4 size film that has been rolled slightly to accommodate the bulging tissue.

8. A patient presents with an extremely large maxillary torus. You are not able to place the periapical films as normal. What should you do?
   A. Move the film to the opposite side of the torus.
   B. Increase the vertical angulation of the film.
   C. Allow the film packet to be lower in the patient's mouth.
   D. Use a no. 0 size film, and take an extra film in the molar area, because all three molars will not fit on one view.

9. To help facilitate correct film placement when the patient has large mandibular tori, the operator should
   A. Use a no. 0 size film.
   B. Place the film less deeply in the patient's mouth.
   C. Place a finger between the torus and the film packet while sliding the film into place.
   D. Place the film on top of the tongue.

10. If a disabled patient is unable to hold a film in his or her mouth, either with a film-holding device or his or her finger, what can the operator do?
    A. Hold the film in the patient's mouth for him or her.
    B. Using an acceptable adhesive, attach the film to the patient's cheek and take a radiograph through the opposite cheek.
    C. Have the patient's parent, guardian, or attendant hold the film after covering him or her with a lead apron, collar, and, if available, gloves.
    D. All the above are acceptable alternatives.

11. When making radiographs on children, the operator should remember that
    A. It is not as important to shield them as it is to shield adults.
    B. The exposure factors may have to be reduced slightly.
    C. It is best to take the radiographs slowly.
    D. It is never wise to tell them what you are doing so that they will not be able to refuse the procedure.

12. The best method to obtain the most accurate endodontic film is to use
    A. The bisecting-angle technique with the patient holding the film.
    B. The paralleling technique with a film holder such as a hemostat or tongue depressor.
    C. The bisecting-angle technique with a film holder such as a hemostat or tongue depressor.
    D. Occlusal radiography.

Chapter 7

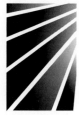

Digital Imaging

INTRODUCTION

Over the next decade, electronic dental imaging, using solid state detectors called **charge-coupled devices (CCDs)** as image receptors, will have a great impact on the clinical practice of dentistry.[1] This filmless "radiography" is already commercially available from several companies (Table 7–1). CCDs are in use in many dental offices inside intraoral videocameras, one of the most widely accepted and successful products using this technology. Although only about 2 percent of U.S. dentists have actually purchased digital x-ray systems at the time of this writing, new products will continue to be introduced. Don't be surprised if you have already used a CCD yourself. If you have sent a fax or own a home videocamera, you have used a charge-coupled device!

Some of the current uses of CCDs follow:

1. Telescopes.
2. Microscopes.
3. Fax machines.
4. Home videocameras.
5. Intraoral videocameras.
6. Intraoral "x-ray" images.
7. Slide and "x-ray" scanners.
8. Panoramic "x-ray" machines.

Intraoral videocameras have been accepted by dentists as a means of improving patient education, disease detection, and treatment-plan acceptance by the patient. Intraoral radiography using CCDs has not yet enjoyed the wide acceptance of videocameras but promises to gain office use dramatically as devices are improved and costs reduced. The important things for you to remember about these systems are that, although CCDs are "high-tech," you still need an x-ray generator to expose this receptor, and the placement of the CCD receptor during image acquisition is identical to x-ray placement with film techniques using a paralleling method. All that really changes is the receptor used to record the information. As more dentists begin to accept both videocameras and intraoral x-ray sensors as a means of improving disease detection and as a way of helping their clinical decision making, the revolution in imaging technology will accelerate dramatically.[2]

TABLE 7–1. COMMERCIAL CCD SYSTEMS

COMPANY	PRODUCT NAME	THICKNESS (mm)	RESOLUTION (lp/mm)	DOSE REDUCTION (VS D-SPEED)
Schick Technologies	CDR	5.0	9–10	80–90%
Trophy Radiology	RVG	6.95	8–10	90%
New Image	NI-DX	8.8	12	90%
Dent-X	Sens-A-Ray 2000	6.0	>15	90%
Cygnus Imaging	CR2	5.0	12	90%

In addition, the acceptance of the computer in the dental office for things like patient billing paves the way for integration of other high-tech tools like digital imaging systems. In the future, image information will become part of the patient's "electronic record," which the dentist will store on a computer disc, compact disc (CD), or other convenient digital storage device.

You're probably asking yourself the following questions: What is digital imaging? How does it work? How will I use it? Read on for the answers.

CHARGE-COUPLED DEVICES AND DIGITAL IMAGING

Currently there are three methods of obtaining a digital image:

1. Direct digital imaging.
2. Indirect digital imaging (digitizing an existing radiograph).
3. Reusable storage phosphor imaging.

Direct Digital Imaging

In the direct and indirect imaging systems, the charge-coupled device (CCD) is used. The CCD is not a new invention; it was developed along with transistors in the 1960s.[3] However, it wasn't until the invention of the computer and fiberoptic image transmission that the CCD became practical for use as an image receptor. The CCD is just a solid state detector—an x-ray, or light-sensitive, silicon chip with an electronic circuit embedded in the silicon. As stated earlier, CCDs are now used in a variety of imaging devices, even panoramic x-ray machines. (Figs. 7–1 through 7–3).

For direct or indirect digital imaging there are two main types of sensor arrays: linear arrays and area arrays (Figs. 7–4 through 7–7). **Linear array detectors** can be placed beside each other in any width. Some prototypes of panoramic imaging

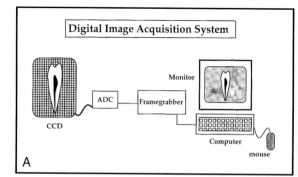
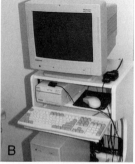

Figure 7–1. *A,* Diagram of a typical direct digital system with CCD (charge-coupled device), ADC (analog-to-digital converter), and framegrabber. The ADC device converts the standard electronic wave to a digital signal by assigning a gray-level number to a spot on the wave curve that corresponds to the signal strength at that point. The framegrabber is an electronic circuitboard that allows the monitor screen to display the image captured by "refreshing" the monitor screen image constantly and rapidly. An x-ray source is still required to expose the CCD. *B,* A typical commercial digital/CCD system.

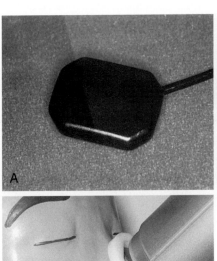

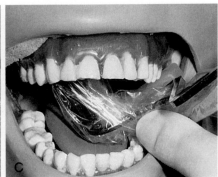

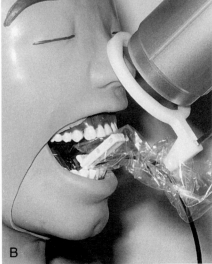

Figure 7–2. A, A contemporary intraoral sensor (NI-DX, from New Image Industries). *B,* Sensor being placed in oral cavity using a PID. *C,* Final position of sensor with cone aligned to PID just as with x-ray film.

systems arrange these linear detectors in a 6 × 12 inch format to approximate the size of a standard panoramic film.

Area array detectors are used with intraoral digital x-ray systems and video-cameras. Although once quite small, area array detectors now have the approximate size of dental x-ray films, both size no. 1 and size no. 2 films. These detectors allow for the acquisition of images in both the vertical and horizontal orientation. Thus, the operator can display a full-mouth series of images.

Note that we refer to "images" instead of "radiographs" or "x-rays" when talking about digital radiology. The digital images are not radiographs, or films, just electronic signals that are captured by CCDs and displayed on computer monitors. Yet they are exposed to x rays to generate the image. "Hard copy" of these images is usually printed on paper. Refer again to Table 7–1 for the currently available commercial systems and their manufacturers. Figure 7–4 depicts each type of direct digital detector, linear and area. Figures 7–5 and 7–6 with their legends describe the process by which the x-ray information is converted into a monitor image for interpretation.

Area array CCDs currently fall into two categories: those that use a scintillator, or intensifying screen, "sandwiched" to the CCD and those that do not. The systems not using a scintillator are termed *radiation-hardened.* Those using a

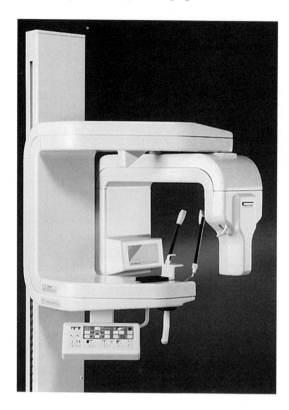

Figure 7–3. The DIMAX digital panoramic machine. (Courtesy of Planmeca, Inc., Wood Dale, IL.)

scintillator (just like a screen/film system for a panoramic or extraoral radiograph) coupled to a CCD include the Trophy and Schick systems. In these systems the x rays strike the screen material and cause photoelectrons to be produced. One x-ray photon will produce hundreds of light photons, which are then gathered in the CCD and transmitted to the computer for processing by a fiberoptic cable (Fig. 7–8).

In contrast, direct, radiation-hardened systems gather x rays directly onto the CCD. Although the image is considered to be more detailed (has better resolution),

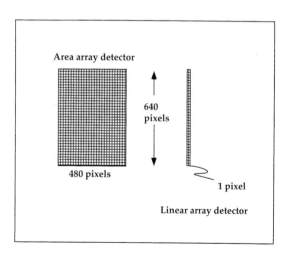

Figure 7–4. Two types of CCD detectors. The area array is used in intraoral videocameras and digital x-ray systems. The linear type array is used in desktop scanners and fax machines.

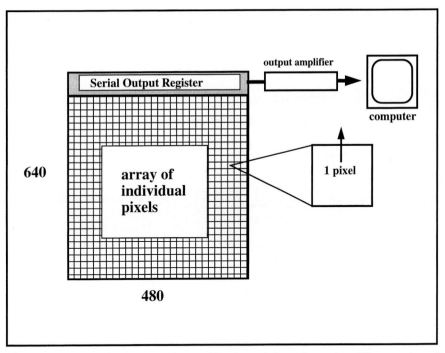

Figure 7–5. Diagram of an area array detector. The electronic image is stored as different numbers of electrons in each pixel. The pixel numbers (values) are read in the serial register as an electric signal strength. The output amplifier enhances the signal for "sampling" by the ADC (analog-to-digital converter) for display on the monitor as described in Figure 7–1A. A typical screen image is 640 by 480 pixels in size. This makes about 307,200 pixels available, each of which can be assigned a different gray level (value). The resultant image is thus highly accurate.

the life of these radiation-hardened systems may be shortened by the direct bombardment of the sensor by the x rays.

Indirect Digital Imaging

Of course, you can "digitize" a radiograph or other document to obtain an image for display on computer. Digitizing is done all the time in the publishing industry. Desktop scanners (lightboxes in which the document or image is placed) capture and digitize the light signal of whatever is placed inside them and are commercially available to anyone (Fig. 7–9). If a dentist wishes to record x-ray film images this way, he or she need only add a "transparency" module to the scanner, which allows the light to be transmitted through the x ray to be recorded. This is like looking at a film on the viewbox, only the lid to the viewbox is closed when the computer program "grabs" the image, digitizes it, and displays it on the computer monitor. Figures 7–10 through 7–12 illustrate the differences between direct and indirect digital image acquisition.

Storage Phosphor Imaging

Storage phosphors are simply reusable materials like those used in intensifying screens to convert x rays to light for detection by a receptor, either radiographic

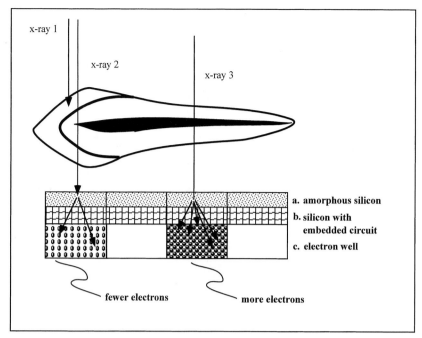

Figure 7–6. Diagram of the interactions of several x rays with a tooth. X ray 1 stops in the enamel; thus, no electrons would be deposited in the CCD in that region. X ray 2 passes through enamel, dentin, and pulp. Upon colliding with the amorphous silicon (a.), covalent bonds are broken (one for each x-ray interaction) and electrons are "kicked out" and attracted to the "potential well." This well is charged positively to attract and hold the electrons. More electrons are created by x ray 3 and deposited in a different well. Each rectangular area of the well region represents a different and separate pixel. Finally, when the electronic circuit (b.) is "opened," the electric signal can be read. See Figure 7–7 for the explanation.

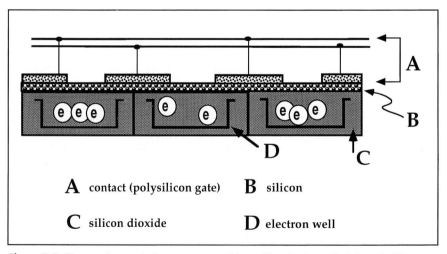

Figure 7–7. Three wells, or pixels, are represented here. The circuitry called the polysilicon gate consists of layers A and B. The electrons stored in the wells (D), embedded in silicon dioxide (C), remain in these wells for only a few milliseconds before the electronic gate is opened to transfer the charge in the well (electrons) to the ADC for conversion to a visible image.

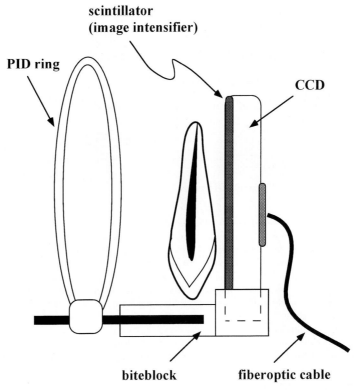

**scintillator
(image intensifier)**

PID ring

CCD

biteblock   **fiberoptic cable**

Figure 7–8. Tooth on biteblock of PID (position-indicating device) with CCD sensor or image receptor ready to receive x-ray information. The wire on back of the CCD carries the image signal to the framegrabber in the computer to view on the screen/monitor. Some CCDs use a scintillator or intensifying screen (as in panoramic cassettes) to amplify incoming x rays and reduce the exposure time needed to produce the image. See Figures 7–10 to 7–12 for explanation of lens versus fiberoptically coupled CCD systems.

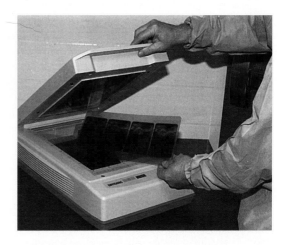

Figure 7–9. A typical desktop scanner that can also be used for digitizing images from paper, slides, or x rays. This is an indirect digital image. See Figure 7–10 for further explanation.

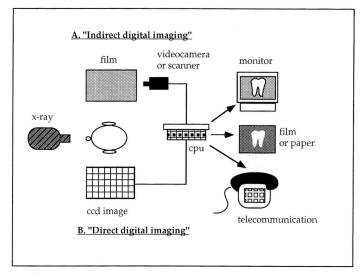

Figure 7–10. Diagram showing film image capture, indirect digital image capture (A), and direct digital image capture (B). When the patient is exposed to x rays using film, the process ends at that point. The x-ray film is taken to the darkroom for wet, chemical processing. The film could also be placed in a scanner or imaged by a videocamera on a viewbox and digitized. This is a form of *indirect digital imaging* because another electronic device has been added to the *imaging chain* to capture the image for display on a monitor. This type of digitization usually is inferior to direct imaging because electronic noise is added to the image, degrading it. A direct capture with an intraoral CCD device as shown in B (direct digital imaging) is preferable. However, once the image has become a digital one in the computer's CPU (central processing unit), it can be (1) displayed on the monitor, (2) printed on film or paper, or (3) sent electronically by telephone modem to insurance carriers or other dentists for remote consultation.

film or CCDs. In storage phosphor imaging systems such as the Digora TM,* an imaging plate coated with the phosphor is used to capture the image. This plate is then placed in a device that uses a laser scanner to read the light signal stored on the plate in the phosphor and display it on a computer monitor. Unlike the CCD, which is attached to the computer by a cable, the reusable phosphor plates have no cable and thus may be placed in the mouth like film. The plate is not as thin as film, but it is thinner than the average CCD receptor. The scanning device adds to the cost of the system, and the plate used for an exposure must be "recycled" to remove the image scanned before replacing it in the mouth for the next view. Therefore, this type of imaging is less rapid than CCD image capture and display. At the time of this writing, reusable storage phosphors appear to be an interim solution for electronic imaging. As CCD receptor systems improve and their cost is lowered, they will replace storage phosphor systems in the dental office. Figures 7–13 through 7–16 depict a typical storage phosphor system.

Imaging Properties and Types of CCDs

As you observed in Figures 7–4 through 7–7, CCDs used in intraoral radiography are arrays of x-ray sensitive pixels. A *pixel* (or *picture element*) is a small "box," or square, into which electrons produced by the incident x-ray or light

---

*Soredex, Helsinki, Finland.

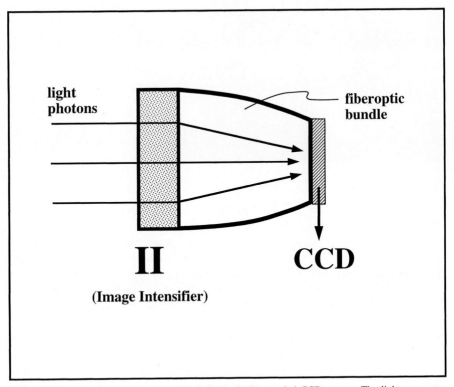

Figure 7–11. This diagram shows a typical fiberoptically coupled CCD system. The light or x rays strike the image intensifier (II), also called a scintillator, and the information gathered by thousands of glass fibers "bundled" together relay the information to the CCD. No information is lost. Compare this with the lens-coupled system in Figure 7–12.

Figure 7–12. A lens-coupled system. Not all the light or x rays strike the lens after interacting in the image intensifier (II). Some are lost. This resultant loss of information makes for an inferior image.

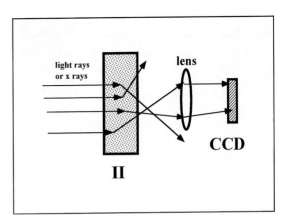

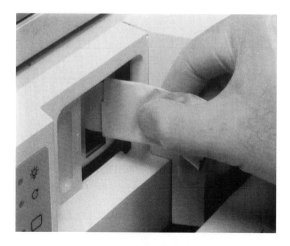

Figure 7–13. A clinician placing a digital storage phosphor. These are small, flexible cassettes with reusable phosphors that store the image as a light pattern until they are read in an optical scanner using a laser beam. The light information is converted by the laser into a readable gray-scale image on the computer screen. (Courtesy of Dr. Robert Langlais, San Antonio, TX.)

photons are deposited (Fig. 7–5). This box, or well, corresponds to a single area (box) on your computer screen as well.

Figure 7–7 is a schematic diagram of electrons deposited in the wells resulting from a direct interaction with the x-ray photons. The x-ray photons have already passed through the patient (these are called the remnant x-rays) and thus indirectly represent the patient's structures, just as a traditional x-ray film exposure would. The legends for Figures 7–10 through 7–12 describe the process of image capture and display.

CCD imaging has distinct advantages over film. This is an electronic system, so the signal can be displayed on a computer, stored on a computer, and subjected to *post-exposure* image processing, including digital subtraction and contrast and brightness alteration. Obviously, you cannot do this with traditional radiographs.

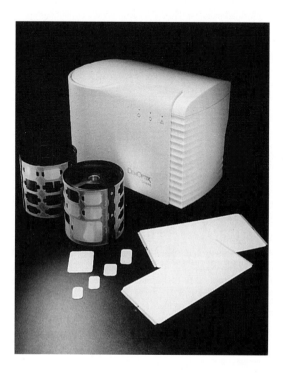

Figure 7–14. An optical scanner that uses a drum to mount the cassettes. Note that the scanner can accept all intraoral film sizes, including occlusal, and that it can also scan a panoramic size image. (Courtesy of Dentsply, Gendex, Milwaukee, WI.)

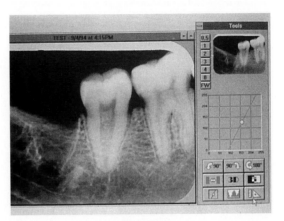

Figure 7–15. Storage phosphor images from a contemporary dental scanner. (Courtesy of Dr. Robert Langlais, San Antonio, TX.)

The digital images can even be sent by videotransmission over telephone lines for consultation or insurance evaluation. This process is termed *teledentistry* by some authors.

Resolution. In imaging, resolution is usually defined in numbers of line pairs per millimeter (lp/mm). Resolution should be high enough to allow you to distinguish between small objects that are close to one another. Dental x-ray film has a resolving power of about 12–20 lp/mm. A typical CCD system is closer to 10 lp/mm. The human eye can resolve only about 8–10 lp/mm. Thus, the CCD appears to have sufficient resolution capability for dental tasks.

X-Ray Sensitivity. The typical CCD sensor is much more sensitive to light or x rays than conventional dental x-ray film. Exposure times for most systems are about 50 to 80 percent less than for E-type x-ray film. Consequently, the absorbed x-ray dose to the patient is substantially reduced with little or no perceptible loss of image detail. A typical exposure time for a digital system for a molar view is three impulses (3/60 s) compared with 12 impulses (12/60 s) for an E speed dental x-ray film.

Wide Dynamic Range. The dynamic range is the digital-imaging equivalent to exposure latitude with x-ray film. For a CCD, the dynamic range is a linear one, and thus the latitude of these systems is extremely wide—greater than that of film. The light, or x-ray, level that is incident on the CCD is displayed by a digital number equal to that amount of energy. Figure 7–17 explains this principle.

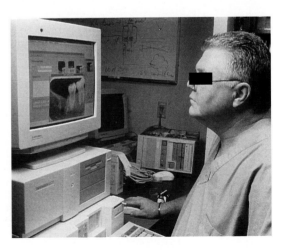

Figure 7–16. Performing an image processing. (Courtesy of Dr. Robert Langlais, San Antonio, TX.)

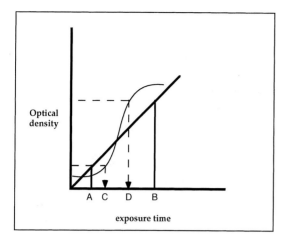

Figure 7–17. Characteristic curves showing the range of useful optical densities produced by two systems: film (curved line) and CCD (straight bold line). Film can be exposed over only a narrow range of exposure times (C–D) compared with the range for a CCD sensor (A–B). This means that the CCD-based systems can portray more x-ray information, especially at either low or high exposures. This quality is called *latitude* in film-based radiography. In CCD imaging it is called *dynamic range*. CCD systems have wide dynamic range.

Photometric Accuracy. Because CCD readout of the electron information is slower than a video camera, each pixel in the array can be digitized with great precision, thus accurately recording the light or x-ray intensity (gray-level) signal accurately. Considering that there are 640 × 480 (or 307,200) pixels in a standard area array detector, each of which can have a gray-level value between 1 and 255, you can see how precise the image-density information can be in these electronic systems.

High Signal-to-Noise (S/N) Ratio. Because the image may be manipulated after the exposure (post-exposure electronic processing), the CCD has a contrast scale similar to that of computed tomography; that is, each pixel can display any one of 256 levels of gray to improve image contrast. This means that a signal—such as an interproximal carious lesion seen as a dark spot on a white enamel background—will be more visible than the surrounding noise in this type of imaging system. Such is not the case with dental x-ray film. Once a film is exposed and processed in chemicals, no more information can be retrieved. Table 7–2 outlines the advantages and disadvantages of CCDs.

TABLE 7–2. ADVANTAGES AND DISADVANTAGES OF CCD SENSORS

ADVANTAGES

1. Instant image viewing.
2. Elimination of the darkroom.
3. Consistent quality.
4. High signal-to-noise ratio (improved detection).
5. Electronic image processing.
6. Greater exposure latitude.
7. Remote consultation capability.
8. Reduced exposure to x rays.
9. Elimination of hazardous chemicals.

DISADVANTAGES

1. High initial cost.
2. Unknown life expectancy of sensor.

TABLE 7–3. POTENTIAL APPLICATIONS OF CCD IMAGING

1. Improved disease detection.
   a. Bone loss.
   b. Periapical lesions.
   c. Interproximal caries.
2. Quantification of disease change over time.
   a. Caries progression or remineralization.
   b. Alveolar bone loss or gain using digital subtraction.
   c. Periapical lesion change after endodontic treatment including apical surgery.
3. 2D/3D reconstruction of the following:
   a. Bone loss.
   b. Implant sites.
   c. Pulp canal morphology (anatomy).
   d. Condylar bone changes.
4. Improved patient education.
5. Remote electronic consultation (teledentistry).

Adapted from Miles DA et al: Imaging using solid state detectors. DCNA 37(4):538, 1994.

Image Applications of CCDs

Clinical tasks such as (1) the early detection of carious lesions, oral cancer, and bone loss and (2) the quantification of any changes in the size of soft-tissue or bone lesions will become commonplace and simple with the use of CCDs. Better treatment decisions will result, all leading to improved patient care. Table 7–3 outlines some of the potential applications of electronic dental imaging for digital x-ray systems. Figures 7–18 through 7–20 show images captured by direct digital CCD systems.

As you can see from Table 7–3, most of the tasks that a dentist is required to perform on a daily basis for patients require some form of imaging. Clinical decision making is based on disease detection by means of correlating signs and symptoms with results of diagnostic tests such as radiographs, biopsies, and so forth. The introduction of these new devices will make these tasks simpler and more accurate for the practitioner. Solid state imaging is here. The sooner dentists adopt this technology into their offices, the more rewarding their practices will become.

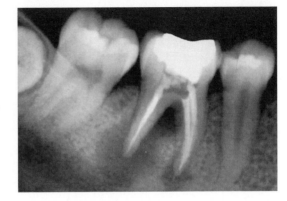

Figure 7–18. Intraoral CCD image.

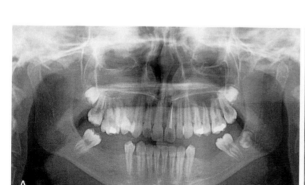
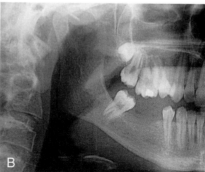

Figure 7–19. A, Panoramic CCD image. *B,* Close-up of patient's right side. (Courtesy of Planmeca, Inc. Wood Dale, IL.)

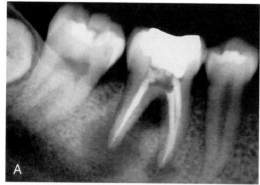
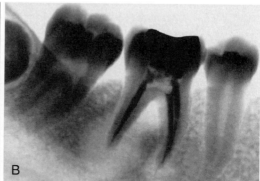

Figure 7–20. Two "processed" images of the same dental image seen in Figure 7–18. *A,* This image has had minor contrast enhancement to see the apical lesions better. *B,* This image has had the contrast "reversed" by the clinician to see the bone in the furcation area between the roots.

References

1. An introduction to the imaging CCD array, Textronix Inc. Technical Note, Beaverton, OR, 1987.
2. Brooks SL and Miles DA: Advances in diagnostic imaging in dentistry. DCNA 37(1):91–111, 1993.
3. Charge-Coupled Devices for Quantitative Electronic Imaging. Photometrics Ltd. Monograph, Tucson, AZ, 1991.
4. Dove B: Digital imaging in dentistry. Newsletter of the American Academy of Oral and Maxillofacial Radiology *19*(1):1,4–10, 1992.
5. Miles DA, Van Dis ML, Razmus TF: Advanced imaging modalities. *In* Basic Principles of Oral and Maxillofacial Radiology, Philadelphia, WB Saunders, 1992.
6. Ramm P: Image analyzers for bioscience applications. Comput Med Imaging Graph *14*(5):287–306, 1990.

Study Questions

1. Methods for acquiring a "digital image" include
   A. Direct CCD capture.
   B. Digitizing or scanning an image.
   C. PSP capture.
   D. A and B only.
   E. All of the above.
2. A CCD is primarily made of the following substance.
   A. Silicon.
   B. Methicon.
   C. Sialastic.
   D. Calcium tungstate.
3. The term "pixel" stands for which of the following?
   A. Picture excellence.
   B. Picture eliminator.
   C. Picture element.
   D. Picture illuminator.
4. All of the following are imaging properties of a CCD *except one.* Which one is the exception?
   A. Precise photometric accuracy.
   B. High signal-to-noise ratio.
   C. High resolution.
   D. Narrow dynamic range.
   E. High x-ray sensitivity.
5. Applications for CCD imaging include which of the following?
   A. Intraoral videocameras.
   B. Panoramic x-ray machines.
   C. Microscopes.
   D. Laser cameras.
   E. Facsimile machines.

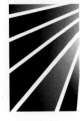

Chapter 8

Panoramic Radiography

*Extra*oral (*outside* the mouth) films, including panoramic radiographs, are taken when large areas of the jaw or skull need to be examined. Small periapical films cannot adequately capture images of the temporomandibular joint, the maxillary sinus, or broad areas of the jaw. Yet, extraoral radiographs do not show details as well as periapical films. Although they are good for evaluating large areas, they are not recommended for detecting subtle changes, such as carious lesions or small periodontal defects.

Extraoral films are often used in conjunction with other dental radiographs for patient evaluation. But sometimes only a film taken outside the patient's mouth will be available for interpretation. For example, obtaining good quality bitewings or periapical films would be very difficult with a patient who is unable to open the mouth wide enough to accommodate these films. In such a case, an extraoral radiograph, such as a panoramic film, may be indicated.

There are many different types of extraoral radiographs. Whereas some of them allow visualization of the entire skull, others focus on smaller areas such as the temporomandibular joint (TMJ). This chapter discusses the panoramic projection. It first describes the equipment necessary to produce panoramic and other extraoral radiographs—cassettes and intensifying screens.

EQUIPMENT

Cassettes

Extraoral radiographs are often made using special cassettes, which are usually flat, rigid, light-tight devices that open like a book. Cassettes keep daylight from reaching the film inside, yet they are made of materials that allow x rays to pass through. They come in various sizes to fit large x-ray films, such as 5 × 7 inches or 8 × 10 inches. Cassettes for panoramic x-ray machines usually measure about 5 or 6 inches in width and 12 inches in length. Panoramic cassettes may be flexible instead of rigid, and they may open at only one end, like a manila envelope (Fig. 8–1*A*). Cassettes must be marked with the lead letters L or R to identify the patient's left or right side, because there is no embossed dot on an extraoral film to tell the front from the back as on intraoral films. Some panoramic units have the L or R built into the head positioner or cassette.

Intensifying Screens

Inside the cassette are two intensifying screens; the film is sandwiched in between them. These screens contain a layer of material called a *phosphor* that can fluoresce, or emit light, when x rays strike it. This is the same material that is used in CCD imaging and is called a "scintillator." It is primarily the light from the screens that exposes the x-ray film. This process acts to intensify, or amplify,

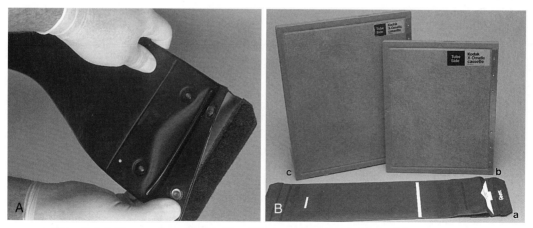

Figure 8–1. *A,* Close-up view of flexible 5″ × 12″ panoramic cassette. *B,* Flexible 5″ × 12″ panoramic cassette (*a*); 8″ × 10″ cassette for lateral cephalometric and other head/neck views (*b*); 10″ × 14″ cassette (*c*).

the action of the x rays; hence, fewer x rays are needed to make a radiograph when intensifying screens are used. The process also results in a film with less resolution, or detail, than a periapical film, because the light from the screens diffuses slightly before exposing the film (Fig. 8–2). The film properties of resolution and detail were discussed in Chapter 4.

Some phosphors, such as calcium tungstate, emit blue light. However, many intensifying screens contain other phosphors that emit green light. These "rare-earth" phosphors are more efficient at converting x rays into light than is calcium tungstate. Therefore, rare-earth screens are "faster" than calcium tungstate screens, and fewer x rays are needed to make a radiograph with them. The result is less exposure to x radiation for the patient.

As mentioned before, the x-ray film is sandwiched in the cassette between the intensifying screens (Fig. 8–3). The film must be sensitive to the kind of light emitted by the phosphor in order for a good image to form. Regular x-ray film is sensitive to the blue light emitted by calcium tungstate screens, but special green-sensitive film must be used with the rare-earth screens.

Film Holders

All panoramic x-ray machines have a special holder for the x-ray cassette. For other extraoral techniques, the patient can hold the cassette, or a mechanical cassette holder can be used (Fig. 8–4). This holder can be attached to the wall, or it can be free-standing. Using a special holder for the cassette is not always

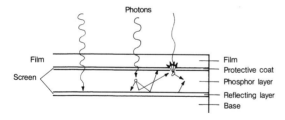

Figure 8–2. One half of a typical screen/film combination. Light striking a phosphor crystal may be scattered or deflected in any direction. Light that "misses" a crystal on its initial passage may strike another crystal after being "bounced" backward from the reflecting layer.

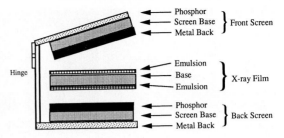

Figure 8–3. A schematic diagram of a typical film-screen combination. Placing the film between two intensifying screens allows for a faster conversion of x-ray photons to light photons. The light exposes the x-ray film much more quickly, and the patient receives less radiation exposure.

necessary, but it minimizes the problem of film or patient movement during the exposure and allows for repeatable exposure geometry.

PANORAMIC RADIOGRAPHY

When visiting the Grand Canyon, one gets a panoramic, or wide, view of the scenery. In radiography, a panoramic film gives a view of the entire maxilla and mandible on a single film. The film is correctly called a *pantomograph* or *panoramic radiograph*. Some people refer to it as a "panorex." Panorex is actually the brand name of the panoramic x-ray machine first introduced to North America by the S. S. White Company in 1959. Unfortunately, this brand name has stuck in the minds of many clinicians as synonymous with a pantomograph.

Today, many types of panoramic x-ray machines are made by different manufacturers (Fig. 8–5). Nevertheless, the basic principles of image formation are the same for most machines. The x-ray tube and the cassette holder are connected to each other across the top of the unit. These components rotate simultaneously around the patient, with the x-ray beam always directed at the film. The area where the images are sharp is a three-dimensional, horseshoe-shaped zone (like the jaws) called the *focal trough* or *image layer* (Fig. 8–6). Only structures in this zone will be clearly recorded; the result is a film that shows the jaws from one side to the other (Fig. 8–7). The rest of the areas of the patient's head are out of focus on the film.

Because each panoramic machine is slightly different, the manufacturer's in-

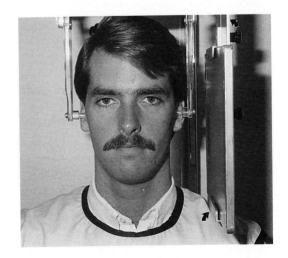

Figure 8–4. Mechanical cassette holder (*arrows*) for a conventional cephalometric unit.

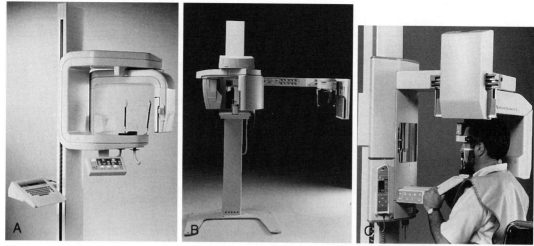

Figure 8–5. Typical panoramic machines. *A,* Planmeca CC Proline with automatic film labeler (imprinter). *B,* Gendex Orthoralix with cephalometric attachment. *C,* Instrumentarium Orthopantomograph OP 100 lowered to accommodate a wheelchair patient. (Courtesy of Planmeca, Inc., Wood Dale, IL; Dentsply Gendex, Dentsply International, Inc., Des Plaines, IL; and Instrumentarium Imaging, Inc., Milwaukee, WI.)

structions for patient positioning and film exposure should be followed carefully. For all machines, the patient should be standing or sitting erect, with the spine as straight as possible. A lead apron that covers both the front and back of the patient should be used. Most of the rotation of the tubehead is around the *back* of the head of the patient. A thyroid collar interferes with a portion of the image and is not used routinely in panoramic radiography. The upward angulation of the x-ray beam minimizes direct exposure of the thyroid gland, a relatively radiosensitive tissue.

The midsagittal plane of the patient's face should be *perpendicular* to the floor, and the Frankfort plane or line of the skull (Fig. 8–8) should be *parallel* to the floor.

The *Frankfort plane* is the line that passes through the floor of the orbit and the external auditory meatus. This plane is sometimes difficult to visualize on a patient. It may help to visualize a line from the ala of the nose to the tragus of the ear

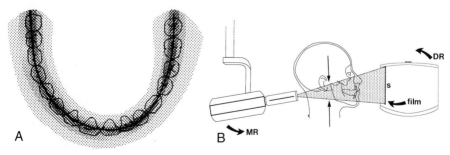

Figure 8–6. *A,* Schematic representation of the focal trough, or image layer, of a panoramic machine. Structures in the middle of the layer will be sharply depicted; those toward the periphery will be less sharply depicted. Outside the layer, all structures will be blurred and magnified. *B,* Diagram shows the "entrance" slit(s) through which the x radiation passes to expose the rotating film. The straight arrows indicate the approximate center of rotation. The curved arrows show the opposite directions of the film versus the machine rotation (*MR*) and drum rotation (*DR*).

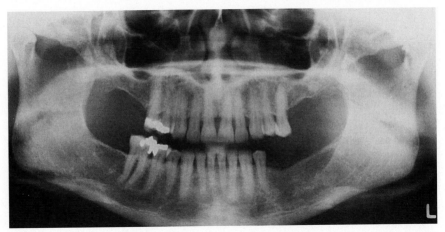

Figure 8–7. A typical panoramic radiograph.

tipped downward about 5 degrees. Some machines position the Frankfort plane automatically for the operator (Fig. 8–9). Many panoramic machines have a chin rest and a bite guide for the patient's incisors. Others have only a chin rest for positioning the patient (Fig. 8–10). Because the focal trough is not a very large area, correct patient positioning is critical in panoramic radiography.

In order to produce a panoramic radiograph of diagnostic quality, several steps must be followed precisely. These include (1) machine preparation, (2) patient preparation, (3) proper patient positioning, (4) proper film exposure, and (5) proper film processing. If any one of these steps is not performed correctly, the subsequent error or errors may lead to a diagnostically unacceptable radiograph.

Machine Preparation

The radiographer must prepare the panoramic machine before positioning the patient. Exposure factors should be selected and set (Fig. 8–11), the cassette should be loaded with an x-ray film and positioned in the panoramic machine holder, and the height of the machine should be adjusted to the approximate entry position of the patient (Fig. 8–12). The operator also should place a sterile bite-pin in the bite-pin holder on the machine (see Fig. 8–9).

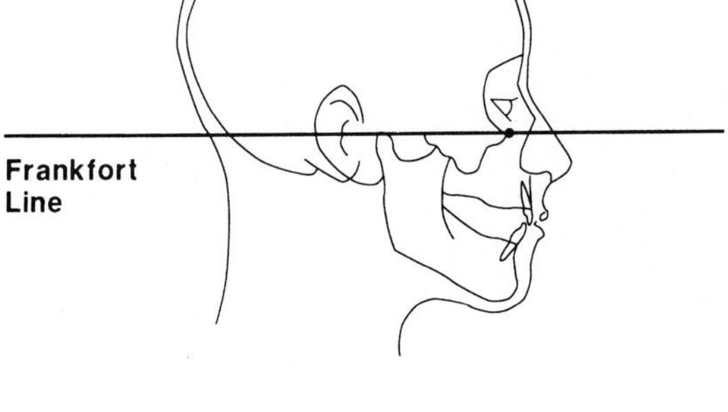

Figure 8–8. The Frankfort plane, or Frankfort line, of the skull.

Frankfort Line

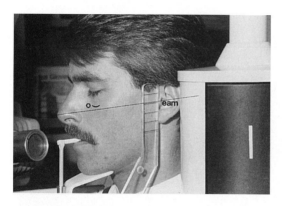

Figure 8–9. The patient's Frankfort plane is correctly and automatically positioned by the machine chin rest because of the chin rest's downward inclination. It is parallel to the linear markings on the head positioner (*arrows*), which also are canted downward approximately 5 degrees. Patient biting correctly on bite-pin. *o,* orbit; *eam,* external auditory meatus.

Patient Preparation

Eyeglasses, earrings, hearing aids, neck jewelry, hairpins, and oral appliances must be removed by the patient prior to the exposure of the film. A lead apron—preferably one that covers both the front and the back of the patient—must be placed on the patient (Fig. 8–13). Instructions to the patient (such as to stand still) or information about the rotational motion of the machine should be given at this time.

Patient Positioning

Proper patient positioning is probably the most important step in the production of a panoramic radiograph. Minor positioning errors can result in artifacts that render the subsequent film at least partially uninterpretable, often in the area of

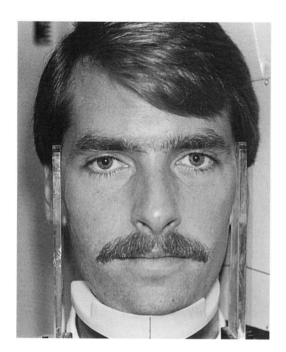

Figure 8–10. A panoramic machine with no bite-pin. A chin rest helps to stabilize the patient's head.

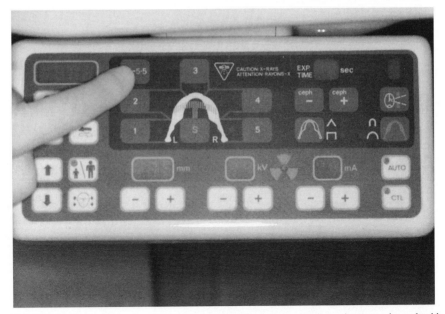

Figure 8–11. The operator is selecting the exposure parameters for the patient on a keypad with microelectronic circuitry. Some views are preprogrammed in the keypad, necessitating that only one button be pushed for those views.

interest. If the film must be repeated, the patient's absorbed radiation dose will be doubled. The operator will also have the embarrassment of explaining to the patient why the repeat film is necessary.

Manufacturers have tried to make the positioning of the patient simple and repeatable. As stated earlier, almost all panoramic machines incorporate a bite-pin

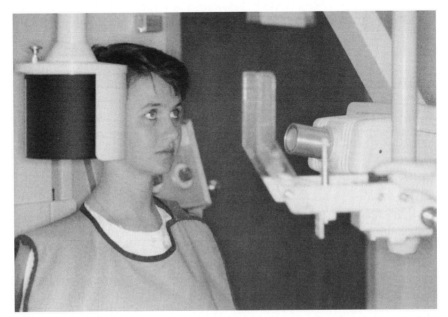

Figure 8–12. The chin rest and head positioner have been "opened" to allow the patient to enter freely.

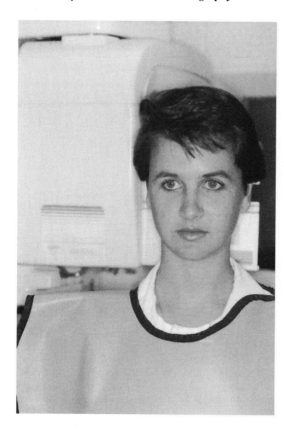

Figure 8–13. A leaded apron that covers both the patient's front and back has been placed on the patient prior to exposure.

(see Fig. 8–9) to position the incisal edges of the central incisors in a region that will result in a diagnostic panoramic film. This optimal region is known by several names, including the *zone of sharpness,* the *focal trough,* or the *central image layer* (see Fig. 8–6). More recent machines have horizontal light guides that demonstrate the occlusal plane or the Frankfort plane and vertical light guides that indicate the correct position of the patient's incisors in an anteroposterior position. These light guides help the operator to center the patient's teeth in the focal trough (see Fig. 8–13).

Generally, for a standard panoramic radiograph, the patient must be positioned with the Frankfort plane parallel to the floor, the midsagittal plane perpendicular to the floor, and the crowns and apices of the incisors centered in the zone of sharpness according to the machine manufacturer's directions.

Panoramic Errors

Schiff and co-workers* studied the most common panoramic positioning errors produced by randomly selected dental technicians, auxiliaries, students, and faculty. These positioning errors are listed in order of frequency of occurrence in Table 8–1. Examples of some positioning errors appear in Figures 8–14 through 8–22.

In addition to the positioning errors described, a number of processing and

---

*Schiff T et al. Common positioning and technical errors in panoramic radiography. JADA *113*(3):422–426, 1986.

TABLE 8–1. FREQUENCY OF PATIENT POSITIONING ERRORS

ERROR	PERCENT	ERROR	PERCENT
Chin low	31.7	Bite guide not used	2
Tongue not raised	25.7	Chin high	1
Patient slumped	12.9	Machine high	1
Head tilted	9.9	Prosthesis left in	1
Head rotated	6.9	Too far back	0
Lips open	4	Chin not in rest	0
Too far forward	2	Patient movement	0

Adapted from Schiff T et al: Common positioning and technical errors in panoramic radiography. JADA *113*(3):422, 1986. Copyright 1986 American Dental Association. Reprinted by permission of ADA Publishing Co., Inc.

technical errors are identifiable by examining the resultant panoramic image. Several of the more common errors appear in Figures 8–23 through 8–26.

Panoramic Anatomy

Interpretation of the many normal anatomic structures, ghost images (both anatomic and artifactual), and pathologic processes imaged on the panoramic radiograph is complicated. As with intraoral radiographs, a sound knowledge of the radiographic appearance of normal anatomic structures or features is mandatory for the operator. Because the production of a panoramic image requires that both the x-ray source and the film rotate around the patient's head, certain anatomic structures—especially those near the center of the patient's head, both external (like the soft tissue of the ear) and internal (like the hyoid bone or spinal column)—will be imaged twice. In some cases structures may even be imaged

Text continued on page 178

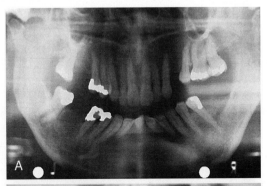

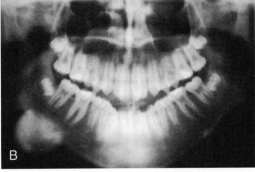

Figure 8–14. A, This patient's chin is tipped down too low. This position causes the occlusal plane to become an exaggerated curve. The lower anterior teeth are positioned farther from the film and are thus magnified and distorted along with the anterior mandible area. *B,* Another example of a patient positioned with the chin too low. The opacity at the right mandibular border is a bony tumor known as an osteoma.

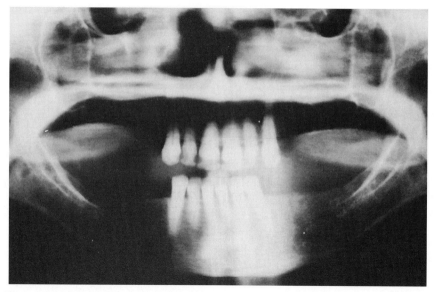

Figure 8–15. An example of a radiograph showing that the patient did not raise the tongue to the roof of the mouth. The black area over the root apices lies between the dorsum of the tongue and the hard palate. These structures will be seen later in the diagrams of normal anatomic structures.

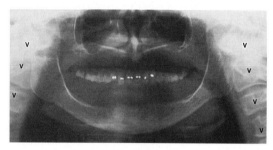

Figure 8–16. This patient was slumped too far forward. The cervical spine was also positioned anteriorly and is projected twice—once on each side of the film (the vertebrae are labeled *v*). Even though the upper denture was left in, the patient had no lower teeth to bite the pin properly. Note also that the patient's tongue did not contact the hard palate, leaving a dark shadow above the denture teeth.

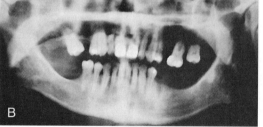

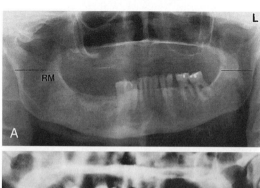

Figure 8–17. *A,* This patient was rotated to the left (*L*). This error caused the right side of the mandible (*RM*) to be farther from the film and thus to be magnified relative to the right side. (Compare the sides and see the difference.) The head has also been tilted, or canted, upward on the left side. *B,* This patient's head was tilted upward on the right side.

174

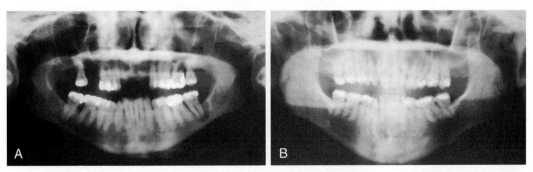

Figure 8–18. *A,* This patient was placed too far forward. Note the slender appearance of the mandibular anterior teeth. *B,* This appearance is even more pronounced.

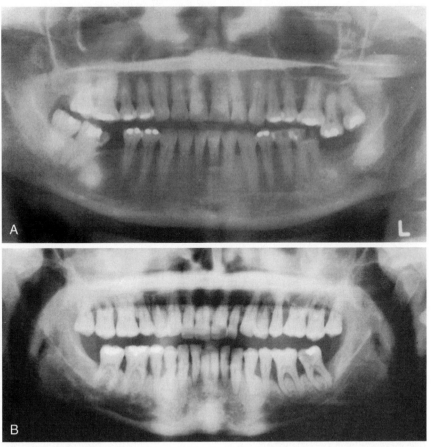

Figure 8–19. *A,* This patient has the chin tipped too high. Note the flattened curve of Spee and the loss of the image of the patient's right condyle. In addition, the patient did not raise the tongue to the roof of the mouth; on the film this resulted in the radiolucent shadow between the roots and the dense radiopaque "band" formed by the hard palate. *B,* Although this patient's tongue was not contacting the hard palate, it obscures information over the roots of the maxillary anterior teeth. (See also the error in Fig. 8–15.)

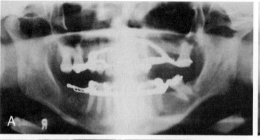

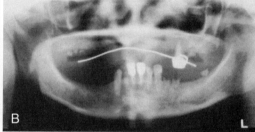

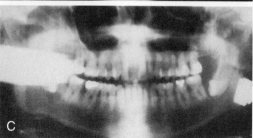

Figure 8–20. *A,* This patient had both a maxillary and a mandibular partial denture left in place before film exposure. This error and the loss of diagnostic information will necessitate an additional radiation dose to the patient, because the film will need to be retaken. *B,* This patient's plastic partial denture was left in place. A thin wire was embedded in the denture's acrylic for strength. Note the wire clasp encircling the maxillary molar for "retention." *C,* This prosthesis is a hearing aid in the patient's left ear. Note the large "ghost" image on the opposite side.

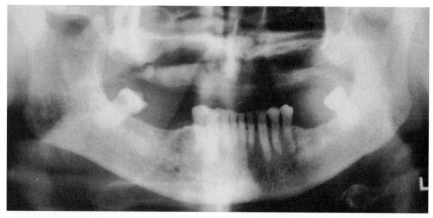

Figure 8–21. The patient's head was rotated to the left. This position resulted in magnification of several of the anatomic structures on the right side, including the mandibular ramus, the permanent second molar, and the hyoid bone.

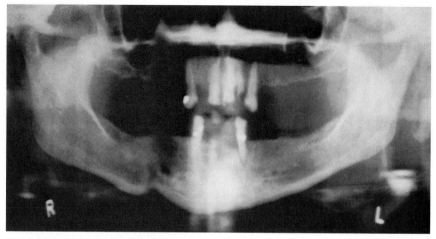

Figure 8–22. The patient moved during the exposure, resulting in an interruption of the image along the mandibular border that resembles a fracture. Note, however, that the distortion extends upward through the entire image to the region of the hard palate. In this film, the patient was also positioned too far forward. Can you recall how you can tell this? (See Fig. 8–18B.)

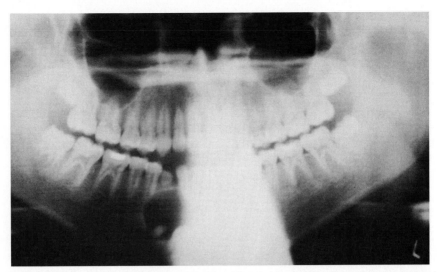

Figure 8–23. The large white (radiopaque) shadow obscuring the images of the anterior teeth—and part of an odontogenic cyst and impacted tooth—was caused by the image of an improperly placed lead apron.

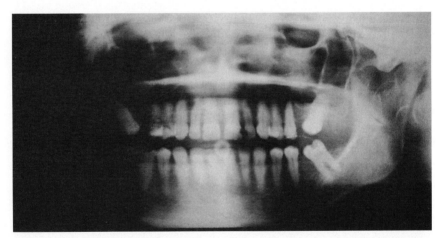

Figure 8–24. The black area on the left side of the film was caused by a light leak. The operator opened the cassette prematurely, when the darkroom lights were still on.

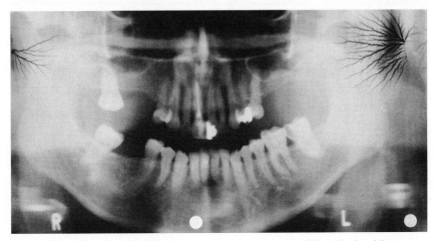

Figure 8–25. These black streaks resembling tree branches were caused by static electricity.

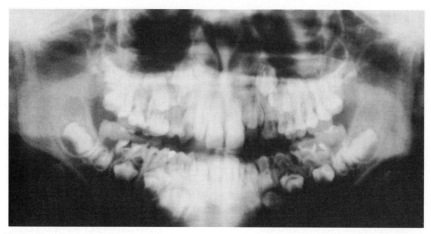

Figure 8–26. The unusual image in this example is the result of a double exposure. The radiographic film was exposed twice in the cassette before processing.

three times. Image formation and image layer formation are beyond the scope of this textbook. An excellent reference for these concepts is provided by Langland and co-workers.*

This chapter is limited to the most common anatomic structures seen on many panoramic films. Not all of these structures appear on every panoramic radiograph every time. However, by studying the legends and by practicing finding these structures on actual panoramic films in your possession, you will become proficient in detecting these normal features so that abnormal features of pathologic lesions will be more identifiable. A diagram is presented in Figure 8–27 to get you started.

*Langland OE et al. Panoramic Radiology, 2nd ed. Philadelphia, Lea and Febiger, 1989.

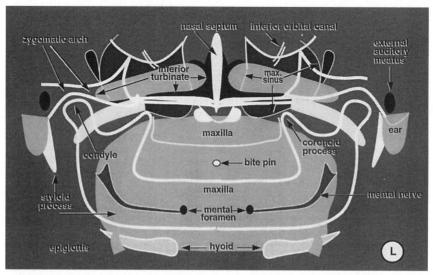

Figure 8–27. This diagram outlines some of the structures that can be visualized on a panoramic radiograph. This example has been labeled with the names of these common structures. Practice naming and identifying these structures before testing yourself on Figure 8–28.

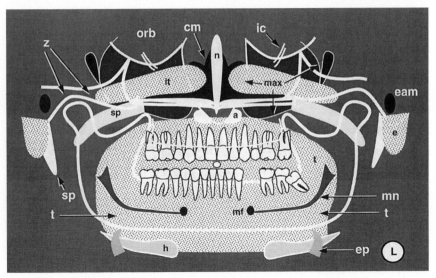

Figure 8–28. See how many structures you can identify without looking at Figure 8–27.

The diagram in Figure 8–28 should be used as a self-test to see how well you have mastered the identification of these structures.

Study Questions

1. Intensifying screens
   A. Contain phosphors that emit blue or green light.
   B. Magnify the amount of radiation.
   C. Absorb scatter radiation.
   D. Are found in the film packets of bitewing and periapical films.
2. The area of the skull that is in focus and thus exhibited on a panoramic film
   A. Is called the latent image.
   B. Is called the focal trough or image layer.
   C. Is called the ghost image.
   D. Is within the Frankfort plane.
3. In general, panoramic radiographs have
   A. Less contrast than periapicals or bitewings.
   B. Greater detail, or resolution, than periapicals or bitewings.
   C. Greater density than periapicals or bitewings.
   D. Less detail, or resolution, than periapicals or bitewings.
4. Which of the following articles would a patient be allowed to wear when having a panoramic radiograph taken?
   A. Earrings.
   B. Necklace.
   C. Wristwatch.
   D. Partial denture.
   E. Hearing aid.

5. You notice a dark streak or band superimposed over the apices of the maxillary teeth on a panoramic radiograph. Which of the following errors occurred during the exposure?
   A. The patient was positioned with the chin too low.
   B. The patient was positioned with the chin too high.
   C. The patient's head was turned to one side.
   D. The patient's tongue was not contacting the hard palate.
6. If a patient was positioned in a panoramic unit with his or her chin too high, which of the following images might be seen on the resultant radiograph?
   A. Narrow, blurry anterior teeth.
   B. Flattened or reversed curve of Spee.
   C. Molars on one side more magnified than on the other side.
   D. Unusually wide anterior teeth.
7. A panoramic film was taken on a patient who had mandibular teeth but wore a complete maxillary denture. You asked him to remove his denture during the exposure. When you looked at the film, the mandibular teeth were very slender and out of focus. What happened?
   A. The patient was positioned too far back in the machine (too far away from the film).
   B. The patient was positioned too far forward in the machine (too close to the film).
   C. The patient's chin was too high.
   D. The patient's chin was too low.

Chapter 9

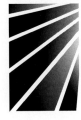

Extraoral Radiography

Making a diagnosis, or assessing a patient's problem, may require information that is not available on standard intraoral or panoramic radiographs. Various extraoral radiographic projections allow the clinician to evaluate specific areas of the skull and jaws that are not included in other types of dental radiographs. This chapter discusses the lateral oblique jaw projections, the cephalometric projections, and the views designed to image the maxillary sinuses and temporomandibular joints. For the most part, these radiographic techniques require rigid cassettes equipped with intensifying screens, such as those discussed in Chapter 8. It is a good idea to label the cassettes with an "L" or "R" marker so that the interpreters know the orientation of the images in relation to the patient. Some views, such as the cephalometric projections, require the use of a cassette holder and a cephalostat to hold the patient's head.

LATERAL OBLIQUE JAW PROJECTIONS

A panoramic x-ray machine can cost three to four times as much as a regular dental x-ray unit. As a result, many dental offices do not have a panoramic x-ray unit. Large areas of the jaw can be visualized without a panoramic unit by using the lateral oblique jaw technique. To perform this technique, have the patient seated and holding his or her teeth together. In the starting position, the patient's occlusal plane should be parallel to the floor with the midsagittal plane perpendicular to the floor. The operator alters the patient's head position slightly as the procedure continues. A 5 × 7–inch or 8 × 10–inch cassette is either placed in a cassette holder or held by the patient between palm and cheekbone, the cassette resting on the shoulder. The cassette is positioned on the side of the patient's face that is to be examined and should contact the patient's cheekbone, ear, and mandible. At least 1 inch of the cassette should extend below the inferior border of the mandible.

Once the cassette has been positioned, the patient should tip the chin up to move the mandible away from the spine. The operator should then tilt the long axis of the patient's head about 15 degrees toward the cassette. This elevates the opposite side of the mandible so that it will not be superimposed on the side being radiographed. If the body of the mandible is the area of interest, the cassette should be in contact with the mandible. The central ray of the beam is directed from beneath the opposite jaw at a vertical angle of approximately −10 degrees to −15 degrees. The beam should be as perpendicular to the cassette as possible, entering in the area of the bicuspids and first molar (Fig. 9–1).

If the ramus of the mandible is the area of interest, the cassette should rest along the cheekbone and the ear. The central ray should be at a vertical angle of approximately −15 degrees to −20 degrees. It should be as perpendicular to the cassette as possible, and it should enter distal to the third molar (Fig. 9–2). Films produced using these techniques should resemble those in Figure 9–3.

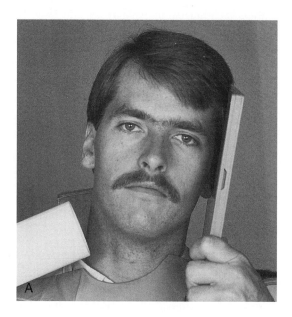

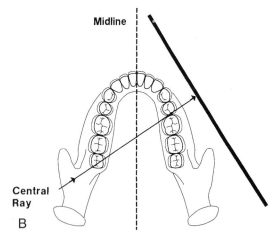

Figure 9–1. *A,* The patient's head and the cassette are angled about 15 degrees from the midsagittal plane. With a negative tubehead angulation of 10 to 15 degrees, the total angle is close to −25 degrees. The thyroid collar has been lowered to prevent its image from being superimposed on the film. *B,* The central ray enters near the first molar for a view of the body of the mandible.

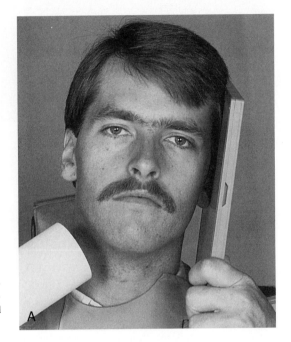

Figure 9–2. *A,* The patient is positioned for a ramus view. *B,* The central ray enters distal to the third molar.

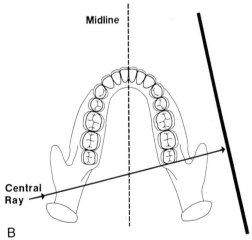

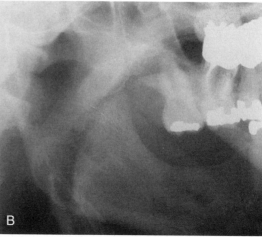

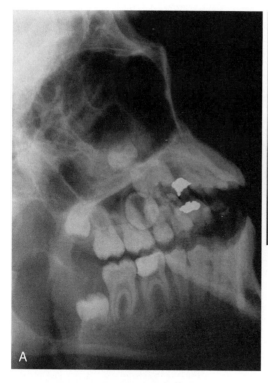

Figure 9–3. *A,* The body of the mandible properly imaged. *B,* The ramus area properly imaged.

CEPHALOMETRIC PROJECTIONS

Some dentists (orthodontists in particular) use a lateral view of the entire skull to assess a patient's profile and to assist in predicting growth patterns of the jaws. The technique is called *cephalometric radiography* (*cephalo* means head, and *metric* means measurement). Because the film is used for measuring arch size changes, it must be taken in a precise manner that can be repeated at a later date.

An 8 × 10–inch cassette is inserted into a cassette holder. The patient's midsagittal plane should be parallel to the cassette, with the left side of the patient's head against the cassette. A *cephalostat,* or head-holding device, helps position the patient by employing rods that fit into the patient's ears. The patient's Frankfort plane should be parallel to the floor. Some cephalostats have a nasion guide that touches the patient at the bridge of the nose to ensure the correct orientation of the Frankfort plane (Fig. 9–4).

The x-ray source is 60 inches from the patient's midsagittal plane in cephalometric radiography. The central ray is directed perpendicular to the cassette, through the long axis of the ear rods. A special cephalometric radiographic unit, in which the tubehead is fixed at the correct distance and alignment, makes beam alignment and patient positioning easy to achieve.

The soft-tissue outline of the patient's profile must be seen on the film in order for you to accurately assess the facial structures (Fig. 9–5). This outline is usually obtained in one of the following ways:

1. By using a thin lead or copper filter at the x-ray source to filter out part of the beam before it reaches the patient's face.
2. By using a wide-latitude, low-contrast film that will record the soft-tissue and bony structures of the head.

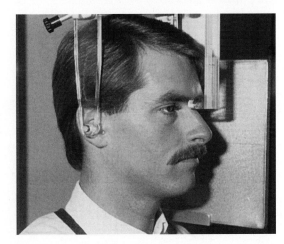

Figure 9–4. The patient is properly positioned with nasion guide in place.

3. By using an aluminum filter strip over the cassette in the area of the patient's profile.
4. By using a cassette with special intensifying screens containing a dye in the area of the patient's profile. The dye will reduce the amount of light emitted from a portion of the screens, and the film will have less exposure in the profile area.

Sometimes an additional cephalometric view is needed to assess a patient's cranial and dental growth and development. A posteroanterior (PA) view is taken with the patient facing the cassette and the patient's Frankfort plane perpendicular to the cassette (Fig. 9–6). The central ray enters at the level of the external occipital protuberance from a distance of 60 inches. A typical film is shown in Figure 9–7.

TEMPOROMANDIBULAR JOINT VIEWS

Imaging of the temporomandibular joint (TMJ) is important to many practitioners, including orthodontists, restorative dentists, and oral surgeons. There are

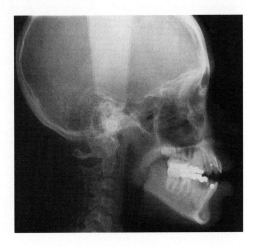

Figure 9–5. A soft-tissue profile of the patient's lips and nose can be seen on this film.

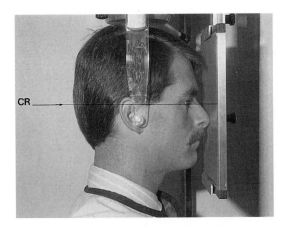

Figure 9–6. Posteroanterior position. *CR* indicates central ray.

many ways to obtain a radiographic image of the TMJ. A standard panoramic film often shows the condyles adequately, although sometimes the glenoid fossa is obscured from view. Some panoramic x-ray machine manufacturers recommend slight changes in both patient positioning and exposure technique to achieve a better image of the TMJ (Fig. 9–8). The procedures for these variations are explained in the manuals that accompany the machines.

Other radiographic procedures also demonstrate the TMJ. A *submentovertex* or *basilar* projection demonstrates the TMJ and other structures as if the viewer were looking upward from under the patient's chin (Fig. 9–9). This view allows the visualization of the condylar heads from medial to lateral poles (Fig. 9–10). Other structures that can be evaluated on this view include the base of the skull, the sphenoid sinus, and, with less radiographic exposure, the zygomatic arches.

Oral and maxillofacial radiologists often use the submentovertex projection in preparation for taking another type of TMJ radiograph, a *tomograph.* Tomographs

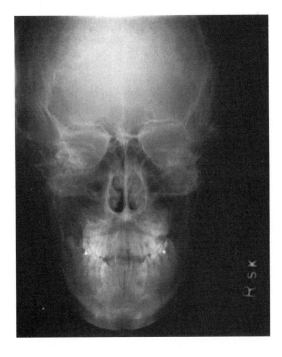

Figure 9–7. Standard posteroanterior view.

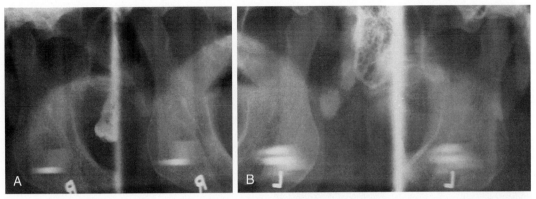

Figure 9–8. A panoramic "four-shot" series of open and closed positions performed on a Gendex Panelipse unit. *A*, Right side closed and open. *B*, Left side open and closed.

must be taken on a special tomographic unit. This machine shows the dentist a "slice" of the joint that is in focus, while "blurring out" surrounding structures. The submentovertex view allows the radiologist to evaluate the position of the condyles relative to other structures and to make adjustments to the tomographic unit so that the tomographic slices are taken in a specific area of the TMJ (Fig. 9–11). Tomographs taken in conjunction with a submentovertex view are referred to as *corrected tomographs.*

Arthrography is a technique for imaging the soft-tissue components of the joint. In this technique, a radiopaque dye (i.e., dye that shows up as white areas on radiographs) is injected into the joint space. The resulting radiographs reveal the condyle, the glenoid fossa, and the joint space, which is filled with dye (Fig. 9–12). Newer tomographic units are computer-controlled and have sophisticated robotic movements. The operator simply selects a program and pushes a button to perform the image acquisition. Figure 9–13 shows one of these units.

In addition to these specialized procedures, several views of the TMJ can be taken in a dental office with a cassette and a regular dental x-ray unit. Procedures for these views are discussed next.

Figure 9–9. The patient should be positioned this way for a submento-vertex projection. The central ray *(CR)* should be directed at an angle of 90 degrees to the cassette.

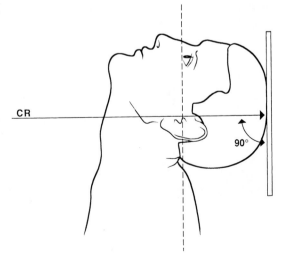

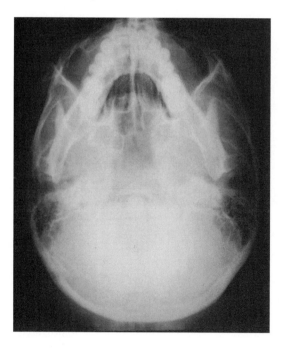

Figure 9–10. Submentovertex radiograph.

Transcranial Projection

There are many different ways to take *transcranial* (i.e., through or across the skull, or cranium) radiographs of the TMJ, but the most common one is the *Lindblom technique.* This technique provides a view down the long axis of the condyle and also shows the glenoid fossa and its relationship to the condyle (Fig. 9–14).

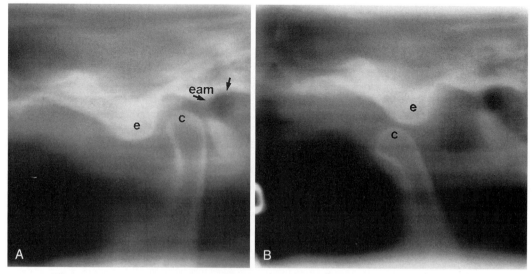

Figure 9–11. Tomographic "cuts" at different depths: *c* is the condyle; *eam* is the external auditory meatus; and *e* is the articular eminence of temporal bone. Each slice is approximately 0.5 cm thick. *A,* View with the mouth closed. *B,* View with the mouth open.

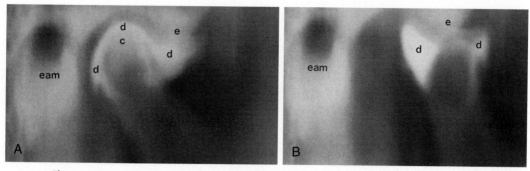

Figure 9–12. Arthrogram of the temporomandibular joint: *c* is the condyle; *d* is the dye; *e* is the articular eminence; and *eam* is the external auditory meatus. *A*, View with mouth closed. *B*, View with mouth open.

The cassette is positioned against the patient's ear and cheekbone on the side being radiographed, with the patient's midsagittal plane perpendicular to the floor. The x-ray beam is directed at a vertical angle of +25 degrees and a horizontal angle of 20 degrees toward the face. The central ray should enter at a point that is ½ inch behind and 2 inches above the external auditory meatus. It is customary to take a view of the patient in both an occluded (closed) and an open-mouth position (Fig. 9–15). It can be difficult to align the patient, cassette, and x-ray beam correctly for this technique. Several commercial devices that assist the radiographer with this procedure are available. These devices also make it easier to repeat the view on a subsequent visit (Fig. 9–16).

Transpharyngeal Projection

A transpharyngeal projection can be obtained quickly and easily, but it does not provide the same view of the glenoid fossa as the transcranial projection, nor is it precisely repeatable. Nevertheless, it can provide an excellent "scout" view of gross changes on the condylar surfaces.

The cassette is placed against the patient's face, in contact with the ear, on the side of the head being radiographed. The procedure begins with the patient's midsagittal plane parallel to the cassette. Next, the patient's head is rotated 7 to 10 degrees away from the cassette. This rotation is made to move the opposite condyle out of the way. The x-ray beam is then directed across the pharynx at a vertical angle of about −5 degrees and at a horizontal angle of about 10 degrees toward the back of the head. The central ray should enter beneath the zygomatic arch on the same side as the tubehead, in the direction of the condyle being radiographed. The patient's jaws may be open or closed. Figures 9–17 through 9–19 illustrate this technique.

Transorbital Projection

The transorbital projection is a frontal type of radiograph that demonstrates the medial and lateral aspects of the condyle, the articulating surface of the condyle, the condylar neck, the articular eminence, and sometimes the zygomatic arch. This projection allows a view that is approximately 90 degrees to the transpharyngeal

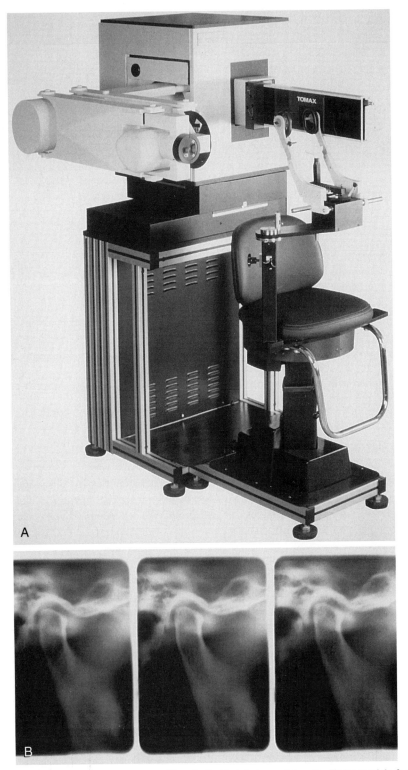

Figure 9–13. A, Contemporary tomographic unit. *B,* Closed views of the mandibular condyle from a tomographic machine. Three views are taken at different depths, or "cuts," from the lateral to the medial poles of the condyle.

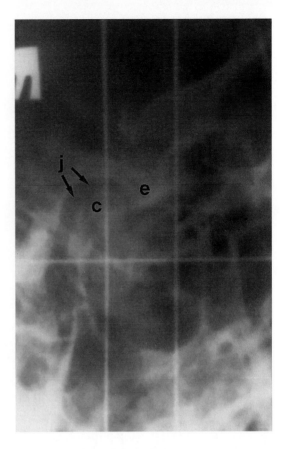

Figure 9–14. Transcranial view of temporomandibular joint: *c* is the condyle; *e* is the articular eminence; and *j* is the joint space.

or transcranial view, usually with little superimposition of other anatomic structures over the areas of interest. The transorbital projection is not a precisely repeatable technique, but, like the transpharyngeal projection, it is simple to obtain.

For this projection, the patient is seated with the Frankfort plane parallel to the floor and the midsagittal plane perpendicular to the floor. The film cassette is placed behind the patient's head on the side to be radiographed. At this point, the cassette should be perpendicular to the patient's midsagittal plane. Without moving the cassette, turn the patient's head approximately 20 degrees toward the side to be radiographed. Direct the x-ray beam at a vertical angulation of +30 to +35 degrees so that the central ray passes through the floor of the orbit and TMJ (Fig. 9–20). The horizontal angulation of the beam should be perpendicular to the cassette. The patient should now open the mouth very wide to move the condyle out of the glenoid fossa and onto the articular eminence. Figure 9–21 shows the resulting radiograph.

MAXILLARY SINUSES

The panoramic radiograph usually provides good visualization of the maxillary sinuses. In fact, the sinuses can sometimes be brought farther forward, into the focal trough or image layer, by positioning the patient 1 cm to 2 cm closer to the film cassette. When an unusual finding is seen in the maxillary sinus on a

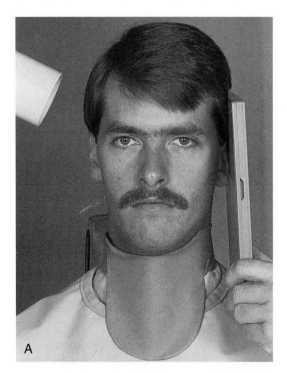

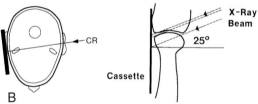

Figure 9–15. *A,* Patient in a position for transcranial radiograph of the temporomandibular joint. *B,* The central ray *(CR)* is pointed approximately 20 degrees toward the patient's face in an imaginary horizontal line perpendicular to the midsagittal plane. A vertical angulation of +25 degrees is customary; consequently, some superimposition of temporomandibular joint structures may be unavoidable.

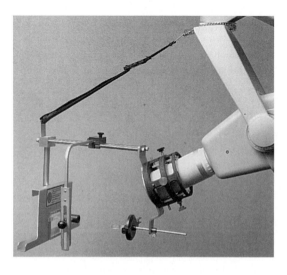

Figure 9–16. A temporomandibular joint x-ray-positioning instrument, the Accurad-200. (Courtesy of Denar Corporation, Anaheim, CA.)

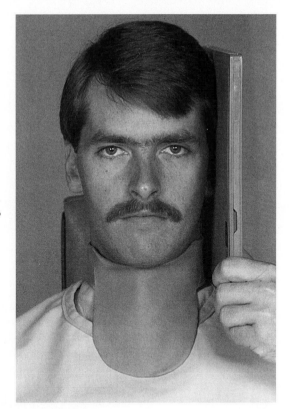

Figure 9–17. *Step 1:* Place the patient's midsagittal plane parallel to the cassette.

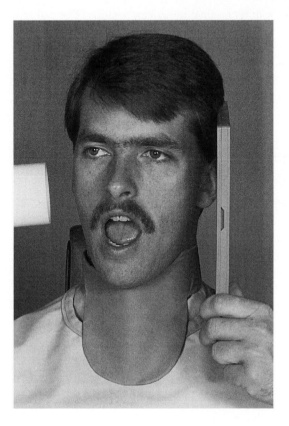

Figure 9–18. *Step 2:* Rotate the patient's head 7 to 10 degrees toward the x-ray source. Open the patient's mouth 35 to 40 mm (a biteblock may be used and the distance measured), and angle the tubehead at −5 degrees in the vertical direction.

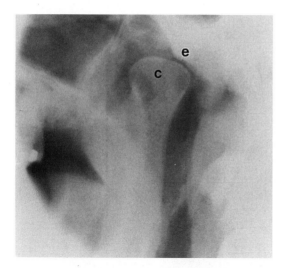

Figure 9–19. Typical transpharyngeal radiograph: *c* is the condyle, and *e* is the articular eminence.

panoramic or periapical radiograph, or if the patient has a complaint in that area, further imaging may be required to reach a diagnosis. The radiographic view that is commonly prescribed for evaluation of the maxillary sinuses is the *Waters,* or *occipitomental, view.* This projection was specifically developed for visualizing the maxillary sinuses. However, the frontal and ethmoid sinuses, as well as the nasal cavity, are also clearly seen on this view.

For this projection, the patient faces the cassette with the midsagittal plane perpendicular to the film. The patient's chin is raised so that the Frankfort plane makes a 37- to 45-degree angle with its original horizontal position. The patient's nose should be 1 to 2 inches away from the cassette (Fig. 9–22). Elevating the chin moves the dense petrous portion of the temporal bone inferiorly on the radiograph, away from the area of interest (Fig. 9–23). Some clinicians prefer to ask the patient to open the mouth during the exposure to avoid superimposing

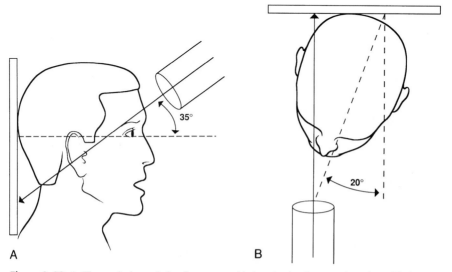

Figure 9–20. A, The vertical angulation for a transorbital projection is approximately +35 degrees. *B,* Rotate the patient's head about 20 degrees toward the condyle that is to be radiographed.

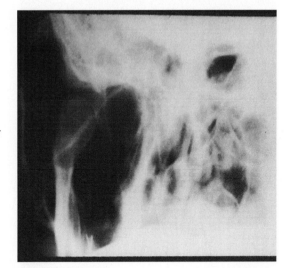

Figure 9–21. Transorbital view of the mandibular condyle.

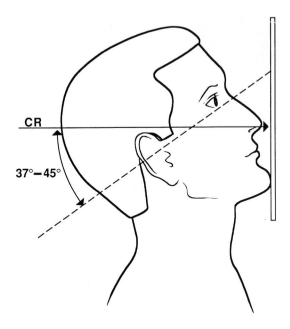

Figure 9–22. For a Waters projection, the patient faces the film and elevates the chin. The central ray (*CR*) is directed at an angle of 90 degrees to the cassette.

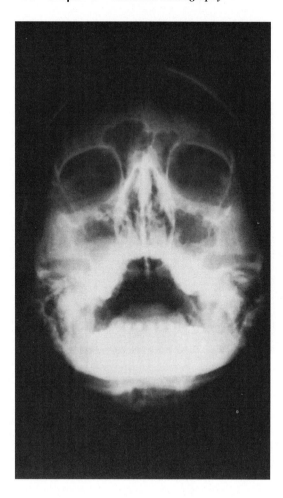

Figure 9–23. Waters view made with the patient's mouth in the open position. The patient's frontal sinuses as well as the maxillary sinuses are demonstrated.

mandibular dental work over the interior aspects of the sinuses. The x-ray beam is directed at 90 degrees to the cassette, with the central ray entering the back of the skull.

Study Questions

1. A lateral oblique or lateral jaw projection may be chosen when
   A. The patient is not able to have an intraoral film, and a panoramic unit is not available.
   B. Views of both sides of the face are needed for comparison.
   C. A view of the mandible without the teeth is desired.
   D. A complete mouth radiographic survey has been taken within the last year.
   E. A soft-tissue outline is desired.

2. A cephalometric radiograph
   A. Is often used to measure changes and predict growth patterns.
   B. Contains a soft-tissue outline.
   C. Is commonly used by orthodontists.
   D. All of the above.
3. A radiographic image that looks like a picture of a skull taken back to front is called a
   A. Cephalometric radiograph.
   B. Posteroanterior view.
   C. Lateral jaw projection.
   D. Pantomograph.
4. The anatomic structures of primary importance on TMJ projections are
   A. The condyle and the coronoid process.
   B. The condyle and the maxillary tuberosity.
   C. The coronoid process and the articular eminence.
   D. The articular eminence and the condyle.
5. A transcranial view refers to
   A. A TMJ projection.
   B. A pantomograph.
   C. A cephalometric view.
   D. A view in one ear and out the other.
6. The technique of imaging a body joint with radiopaque dye is called
   A. Cephalometrics.
   B. Tomography.
   C. Arthrography.
   D. The submentovertex technique.
7. The TMJ view that allows you to see the medial and lateral aspects of the condyle is the
   A. Transorbital projection.
   B. Transcranial projection.
   C. Transpharyngeal projection.
   D. Waters projection.
8. A radiographic technique for evaluation of the maxillary sinuses is the
   A. Submentovertex view.
   B. Transcranial view.
   C. Transorbital view.
   D. Waters view.
9. Which pair of radiographs would appear to be similar to each other?
   A. Submentovertex and panoramic views.
   B. Transcranial and transorbital views.
   C. Transcranial and transpharyngeal views.
   D. Transpharyngeal and submentovertex views.
   E. Submentovertex and Waters views.

Chapter 10

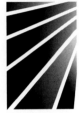

Implant Radiology

INTRODUCTION

Implant procedures are now commonplace in the dental office. General dentists use root form implants, not just dental specialists.[1, 3] Presurgical radiographic evaluation of endosseous, or root form, implants is central to the success of the implant procedure. This chapter reviews various imaging modalities, from intraoral radiographs to computed tomography (CT) imaging, to give the clinician and auxiliary personnel a better understanding of which imaging techniques are best suited for evaluating various implant sites. The technique for placement of the films for implant assessment is no different than standard intraoral periapical technique with this exception: a precise paralleling method is mandatory for eliminating errors of vertical angulation inherent in the bisecting-angle technique, a technique that is inappropriate for implant site assessment.

The success of any surgical implant procedure lies partly in the preoperative planning.[3] Case selection involves both the clinical assessment of the site(s) by visual examination, and *appropriate* radiographic imaging.[2, 4–8] Other factors include patient education, patient preparation, and risk estimation for the procedure. We will confine our discussion here to the selection of the appropriate imaging procedure for endosseous, or root form, implants. The role of radiography in the presurgical phase will be outlined, as well as the advantages and limitations of each imaging modality.

PERIAPICAL, OCCLUSAL, AND PANORAMIC TECHNIQUES

Presurgical radiographic evaluation of implant sites should help the dentist determine

1. The quantity of bone present.
2. The quality of bone available.
3. The location of critical anatomic structures.

Generally, it is sound practice to obtain multiple views of the proposed site to adequately assess the height and width of the bone. This assessment may require several imaging techniques.[1, 3]

For a single site it is advisable to take several periapical radiographs and at least one properly positioned and exposed occlusal radiograph. These films afford the best image detail of a single site with minimal geometric distortion. Intraoral radiographs are useful to help determine the approximate height of the bone as well as the distance of the proposed site from important anatomic structures such as the mental foramen, the maxillary sinus, the inferior alveolar nerve, and the incisive and canine fossae (Figs. 10–1 through 10–3).

An occlusal film taken at 90 degrees to the mandibular dental arch gives excellent information about the buccolingual width of the bone (Fig. 10–4). But the shape, or architecture, of the bone in three dimensions is not always apparent

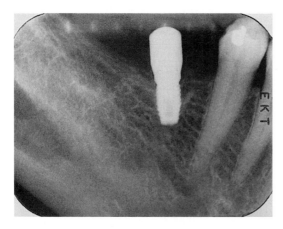

Figure 10–1. Important structures such as the mental foramen are best visualized in the sagittal plane by detailed intraoral periapical films. These are then correlated with panoramic and tomographic views.

Figure 10–2. This implant was positioned well away from the maxillary sinus floor.

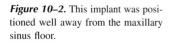

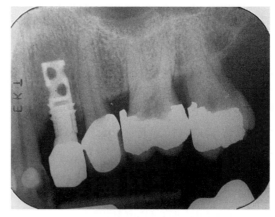

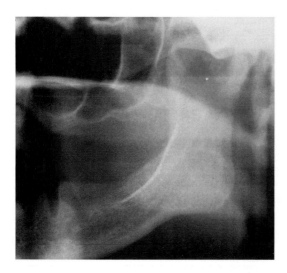

Figure 10–3. A panoramic radiograph is an excellent scout film to view the morphology of the maxillary sinuses bilaterally. Here there is obviously no bone for a fixture unless a surgical procedure such as a sinus augmentation or sinus lift is performed beforehand.

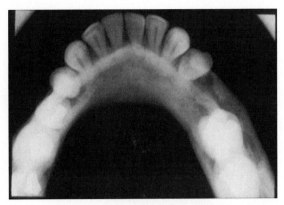

Figure 10–4. A mandibular occlusal view to help determine the buccolingual width.

on an occlusal film, especially in the posterior mandible (Fig. 10–5). An occlusal view of the maxilla is often distorted and hence may be less useful for arch width determination (Fig. 10–6). Additional views, such as tomographs, may be required for adequate assessment.

Intraoral films, together with panoramic radiographs, can reveal information about bone quality such as density and trabecular pattern and about the presence of anomalies in the proposed region. Additionally, panoramic radiographs, if properly positioned, are useful adjuncts for even single implant site selection because they allow comparison with contralateral structures. Panoramic films are also useful for a preliminary look at multiple implant sites (Fig. 10–7). **Nevertheless, panoramic radiology as the sole means of radiographic presurgical assessment is inappropriate, because the technique is extremely sensitive to errors in patient position. Several authors have outlined these errors and their correction.**[2, 7]

Many articles in the literature contain pre- and postoperative panoramic radiographs showing distortion resulting from one *or more* positioning errors. If clinicians continue to use only this imaging technique for implant assessment, they must be sufficiently trained in panoramic radiology to understand its limitations. If not, they risk potential litigation problems owing to inadequate radiographic assessment that may contribute to failure of the procedure.

In addition to the myriad of possible positioning errors, the use of panoramic

Figure 10–5. CT reconstruction of an edentulous mandible showing a large depression, the submandibular fossa.

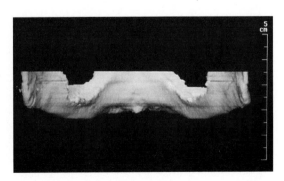

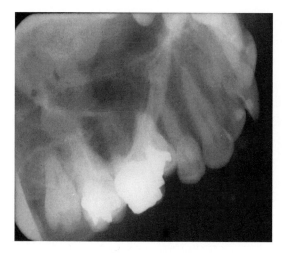

Figure 10–6. A maxillary occlusal view of the upper left side of the patient. Note how the sinus and zygoma overlap the bone and teeth. This type of view could not be used for determining implant site width.

films alone may lead to errors in estimating or determining the bone width. Several other imaging modalities, such as tomography and computed tomography, give better information on the anatomy of the proposed site, which can help the clinician avoid potential problems. Figures 10–8 through 10–10 demonstrate typical errors in panoramic imaging of implant sites.

INTRAORAL IMAGING USING ELECTRONIC OR CCD IMAGING TECHNIQUES

Now that dentists are beginning to use charge-coupled devices (CCDs), presurgical implant assessment of single sites may become more precise. These area array, solid state detectors called CCDs were described in Chapter 7. They allow a more accurate measurement of implant sites preoperatively and provide more information about osseointegration postoperatively than has been available with film. Image processing techniques such as measurement tools help clinicians with site selection and bone height determination and are contained in most manufacturers' accompanying software.

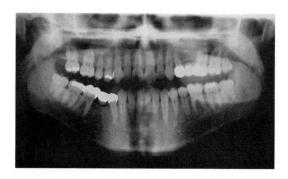

Figure 10–7. A reasonably well-positioned and well-exposed panoramic radiograph.

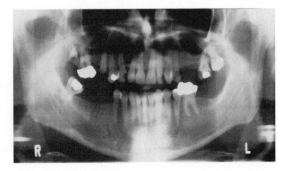

Figure 10–8. Patient is positioned too far forward, distorting the anterior teeth. The chin may also be tipped too far down, which will result in an overestimation of true bone height in the posterior region.

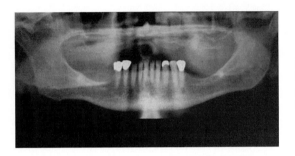

Figure 10–9. The patient's chin here is too far up. The bone height in the molar regions may actually be better or higher than the film suggests.

Figure 10–10. This patient's head has been rotated to the left, making the right body and ramus of the mandible appear larger. The film is thus useless for measuring bone height.

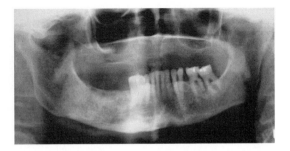

As computers are integrated more into the imaging process, software will be developed to use multiple images of a proposed site to construct two- and three-dimensional pictures for the dentist to view on a computer screen. The result would be similar to that of current CT imaging but with less expense.

TOMOGRAPHIC TECHNIQUES

For fewer than three proposed implant sites, the most cost-effective method of radiographic assessment is probably plain film tomography. *Plain tomography* refers to the simultaneous movement of the x-ray tube and x-ray film in opposite directions to produce a "slice," or selected image layer, in which there is increased contrast (resolution) showing details of the structures of interest.

In linear tomography the film and x-ray tube pass in opposite directions, in a horizontal or vertical manner, through an imaginary fulcrum that represents the image plane (Fig. 10–11). The "slice" thickness generally varies from 3 to 5 mm with linear machines. The image layer may be narrower for multi- or pluridirectional units that travel through more complex movements. Figures 10–12 and 10–13 show examples of films of various implant sites using several commercially available machines.

COMPUTED TOMOGRAPHY (CT)

Computed tomography (CT), with its two-dimensional and three-dimensional reconstruction capability, is probably the most useful and precise imaging modality

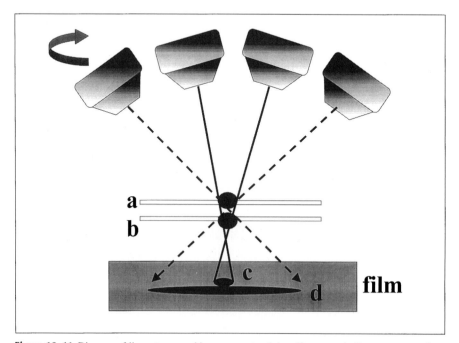

Figure 10–11. Diagram of linear tomographic movement and the effect on a similar structure at plane *a* and plane *b*. Note that the object shadow *d* at plane *b* has a much wider and more distorted appearance than the object c from plane *a*.

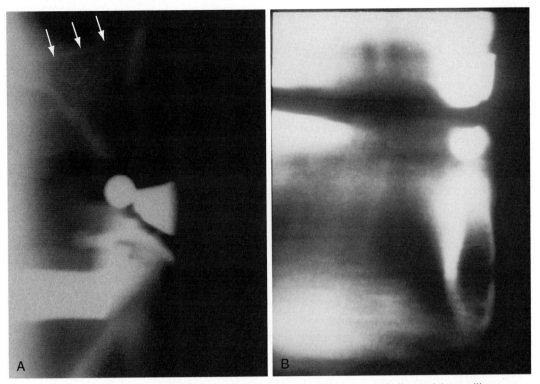

Figure 10–12. *A*, Proposed implant site in anterior maxilla. Note how symmetrically round the metallic ball is. This means that there is no distortion. The arrows point to the floor of the nasal fossa. *B*, Mandibular tomograph of proposed site in posterior region.

Figure 10–13. Another mandibular site. Note the prominent appearance of the mental foramen. There appears to be both adequate width and height for an implant fixture here.

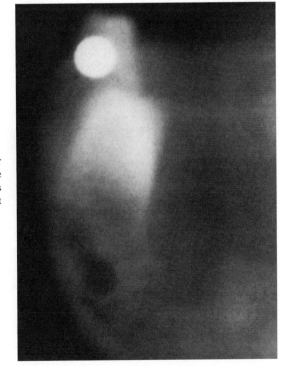

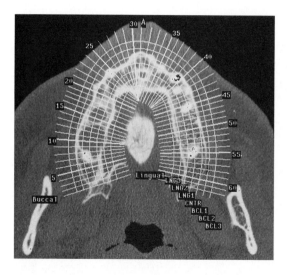

Figure 10–14. This is an axial view of a section of the maxilla at the level of the mid palate. The large opacity in the middle of the palate is a maxillary torus. See if you can pick out the sinus spaces (hint: they appear as radiolucent circles intersected by the tangent line markings 10 and 15). See if you can pick out roots of teeth as well. Remember, the roots are seen in this axial view in cross section. They would appear as rounded radiopaque structures!

for presurgical assessment. If multiple sites in the maxilla, mandible, or both are being evaluated or proposed, CT may even be the most cost-effective technique. Plain tomographic imaging of multiple sites is quite labor-intensive, and thus the fees tend to be much higher than for one or two sites. Another advantage of CT over plain tomography is that most contemporary workstations and software used to process the CT image data are rapid, detailed, and allow visualization of the proposed sites on a 1:1 ratio—that is, life-sized.

Figures 10–14 through 10–16 demonstrate the information available from such examinations. Three-dimensional visualization as seen in Figures 10–17 and 10–18 represents the state of the art in imaging techniques at the time of this writing. Because the most appropriate approach to a successful implant is multidisciplinary, the assistance of a medical or oral and maxillofacial radiologist is appropriate, as they can also evaluate the tomographic and CT images for problems other than those associated directly with the implant assessment.

Table 10–1 summarizes the application(s), usefulness, and limitations of all the techniques discussed here for use in the presurgical evaluation.

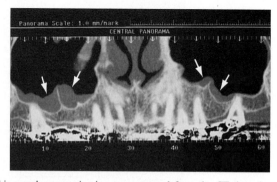

Figure 10–15. This pseudopanoramic view reconstructed from the CT data shows a "slice" of the patient's maxilla from side to side in the middle of the maxillary bone. You should be able to make out root structures and the sinus floors. The gray shadows above the sinus floors (*arrows*) represent thickening of the lining mucosa of the sinuses. This patient has either allergies or a low-grade sinus inflammation or infection.

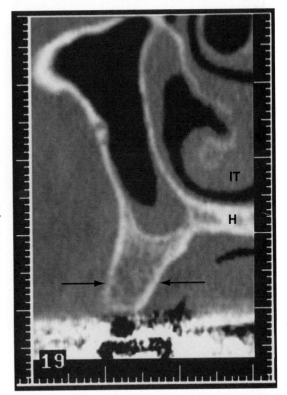

Figure 10–16. This is a close-up view of the maxilla in the bicuspid/premolar region as seen in a coronal section (patient sliced from front to back). You can still see the soft tissue in the sinus. *H* is the hard palate; *IT* is the inferior turbinate bone. The bone width available lies between the arrows.

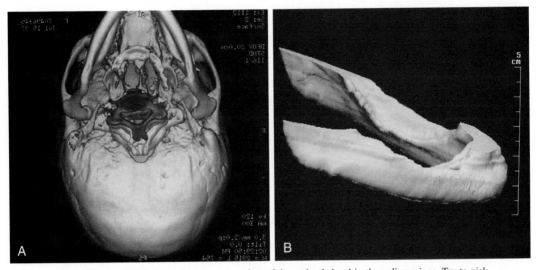

Figure 10–17. A, This is a submentovertex view of the patient's head in three dimensions. Try to pick out the condyles of the mandible. Then challenge yourself to find other anatomic structures you might recognize. *B,* This is a partial 3D view of the mandible showing greater height in the anterior region between the former cuspid area. See if you can find the mental foramen. Figure 10–5 is the same patient shown from a different angle.

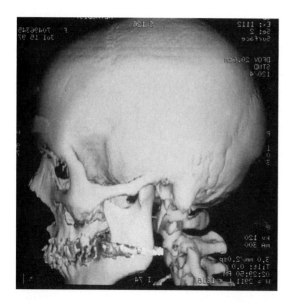

Figure 10–18. This is the same patient as viewed in three dimensions from the side. Pick out the condyles, zygomatic arch, and mastoid process, as well as other structures you recognize.

TABLE 10–1. IMPLANT IMAGING—PRESURGICAL ASSESSMENT

EXAM TYPE	APPLICATION	USEFULNESS	LIMITATIONS
Periapical	Single implant site	Good detail. Minimal geometric distortion.	Small size. Two-dimensional only, not three-dimensional. Hard to reproduce after placement. Little anatomy visible.
Occlusal	Single implant site	Good detail. Buccolingual dimensions. Larger area of coverage.	Little anatomy visible. Distortion in maxilla owing to technique.
Panoramic	Multiple sites General view of bone, anatomy	Can see anatomic structures such as foramina, sinuses, etc.	Less detail. Geometric magnification. Positioning errors likely unless sufficient technique training.
Tomography	Exact imaging of implant site	Very useful, detailed view of implant site(s). Little superimposition of other anatomic structures.	Equipment cost. Trained oral radiologist must be available to perform the procedures and calculate bone dimensions.
CT	Imaging of multiple implant sites	Precise estimation of available bone levels. Automatic calculation of bone height and width. Reconstruction of image is possible.	Equipment cost. Software must be available at hospital radiology service. Access must be provided to CT unit.

Adapted from Miles DA and Van Dis ML: Implant Radiology. DCNA 37(4):645–668, 1993.

References

1. Kassebaum DK, Nummikoski PV, Triplett RG, and Langlais RP: Cross-sectional radiography for implant site assessment. Oral Surg 70:674, 1990.
2. Langland OE, Langlais RP, McDavid WD, and DelBalso AM: Troubleshooting errors in panoramic techniques. *In* Panoramic Radiology, 2nd ed., Philadelphia, Lea and Febiger, 1989.
3. McKinney RV Jr: Evaluation and selection of the endosteal implant patient. *In* Endosteal Dental Implants, St. Louis, Mosby–Year Book Inc., 1991.
4. Miles DA, Van Dis ML, and Razmus TF: Advanced imaging modalities. *In* Basic Principles of Oral and Maxillofacial Radiology, Philadelphia, WB Saunders, 1992.
5. Poon CK, Barss TK, Murdoch-Kinch CA, Bricker SL, Miles DA, and Van Dis ML: Presurgical tomographic assessment for dental implants: Part 1. A modified imaging technique. Int J Oral Maxillofac Implants 7:246, 1992.
6. Schwarz MS, Rothman SLG, Rhodes ML, and Chafetz N: Computed tomography: Part 1. Pre-operative assessment of the mandible for endosseous implant surgery. Int J Oral Maxillofac Implants 2:143,1987.
7. Schiff T, D'Ambrosio J, Glass BJ, Langlais RP, and McDavid WD: Common positioning and technical errors in panoramic radiography. JADA 113:422,1986.
8. Tal H and Moses O: A comparison of panoramic radiography with computed tomography in the planning of implant surgery. Dentomaxillofac Radiol 20:40,1991.

Study Questions

1. Presurgical implant radiographs are taken for each of the following reasons *except one*. Which one is the exception?
   A. To determine bone quantity.
   B. To locate anatomic structures.
   C. To find areas of bone density.
   D. To assess the quality of bone.
2. Radiographic techniques that allow a dentist to view a proposed implant site in the "third" dimension or plane include
   A. Occlusal film.
   B. Plain tomography.
   C. Computed tomography.
   D. Panoramic radiology.
   E. CCD imaging.
3. Which of the following radiographic techniques is most susceptible to errors of position?
   A. Panoramic radiology.
   B. Linear tomography.
   C. Intraoral periapical technique
   D. Computed tomography.
4. Which of the following techniques provides the best "detail" or resolution for a proposed implant site?
   A. Intraoral periapical technique.
   B. Panoramic radiology.
   C. Plain tomography.

5. Which of the following are limitations of computed tomography for implant assessment?
   A. Availability of implant software.
   B. Access to a scanner.
   C. Availability of a radiologist trained to process these images.
   D. Cost of the equipment.
   E. A, B, and C.
   F. All of the above.

Chapter 11

Normal Anatomy and Film Mounting

The knowledge of normal anatomic landmarks is indispensable to the dental auxiliary, because it is this knowledge that facilitates the mounting of radiographs in their proper location and sequence. An error in film mounting could result in improper treatment of the dental patient. This chapter assumes that the student has already received instruction in basic anatomy, including the bony anatomy of the maxilla and the mandible. The student must be able to identify normal anatomic landmarks in the maxilla and the mandible on radiographs in order to be able to detect abnormal findings. Normal structures encountered on dental radiographs can sometimes resemble pathologic areas. This chapter identifies the common radiographic anatomic landmarks seen on the intraoral films. Not all of the structures identified appear each time on each film. The images on dental radiographs vary widely, owing to differences in technique as well as in patient anatomy. Chapter 12 compares normal anatomy with certain pathologic conditions that may have similar radiographic presentations.

Many of the illustrations in this chapter repeat landmarks. This is to reinforce your learning. The structures vary in appearance depending on the angulation of the film or the tubehead. Some of the illustrations in this chapter also have questions for you to answer; a figure reference to remind you of the answer often follows the questions. Finally, instructions for mounting radiographs based on anatomic landmarks are included at the end of this chapter.

TEETH AND ADJACENT STRUCTURES

The Tooth

Enamel, dentin, cementum, and pulp tissue are the components of a tooth. Of the four tissues, enamel is the hardest. Next are the dentin and cementum. The pulp tissue is soft tissue and thus is not visible on the radiograph but is represented by a dark space within the tooth (Fig. 11–1). In contrast, the enamel appears white on the film. It is very dense and attenuates (stops) more x rays than the other dental tissues; it can therefore be easily distinguished from the dentin. A distinct and often abrupt interface between enamel and dentin in the crown, or coronal portion, of the tooth is called the *dentinoenamel junction* (DEJ). The DEJ is apparent in Figure 11–1.

Dentin is less dense than enamel but has a density similar to both cementum and bone. The cementum is a thin layer of tooth structure that covers the entire root surface. The interface between the dentin and the cementum in the root portion of the tooth is not visible radiographically. The radiographic density of dentin and cementum is between that of the white enamel and the black pulp space and therefore appears gray.

Bone, Periodontal Ligament Space, and Lamina Dura

Bone, like dentin, is usually less dense than enamel and therefore usually appears gray on radiographs. Bone supporting the teeth appears as irregularly

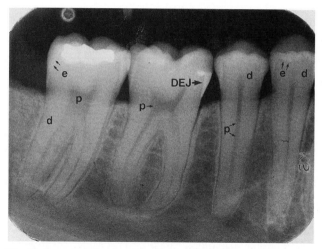

Figure 11–1. Mandibular periapical radiography: dentin *(d)*, enamel *(e)*, pulp space *(p)*, and dentino-enamel junction *(DEJ)*.

shaped lines in random patterns called *trabeculae* that surround marrow spaces. The trabecular pattern of bone is extremely variable; even normal variations can look very different from one another. This type of bone is called *cancellous bone*.

Cortical bone is bone without marrow spaces and thus is usually more dense and more distinct than cancellous bone. Examples of cortical bone are the crests of the alveolar process and the lamina dura. The alveolar process itself consists of the cortical crests, the cancellous bone, and the lamina dura. On occasion, the bone referred to as the lamina dura can be relatively dense, or white, similar to enamel (Fig. 11–2).

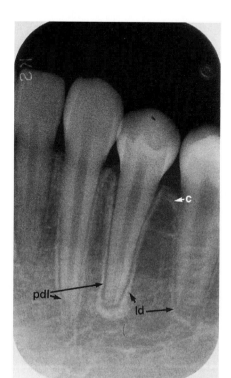

Figure 11–2. Periodontal ligament *(pdl)*, the thin radiolucent line adjacent to the root surface; lamina dura *(ld)*, the white radiopaque line between the *pdl* and the cancellous bone; and cortical bone *(c)*, in this example the alveolar crest.

The periodontal ligament (periodontal membrane), like the pulp tissue, is not visible on the radiograph. However, the space it occupies is apparent. It is therefore termed the *periodontal ligament space* or *periodontal membrane space*. It appears on a radiograph as a *continuous* dark line around the root of the tooth from one interproximal area to the next (Fig. 11–2).

When healthy, both the periodontal ligament space and the lamina dura are continuous around the root. The lamina dura is also continuous with the alveolar ridge crest (crestal cortex). Figures 11–1 and 11–2 demonstrate this.

MAXILLARY ANATOMIC LANDMARKS

Figures 11–3 through 11–26 identify various maxillary anatomic landmarks and, in some instances, invite the reader to identify them.

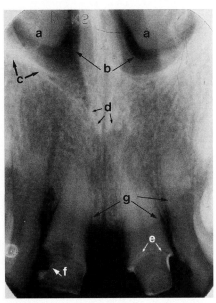

a. Inferior turbinate bone.
b. Inferior meatus.
c. Lateral wall of nasal fossa.
d. Anterior nasal spine.
e. Crown preparation.
f. Carious lesion or nonradiopaque filling material.
g. Shadow of the nose (soft-tissue outline).

Figure 11–3. Central incisor view.

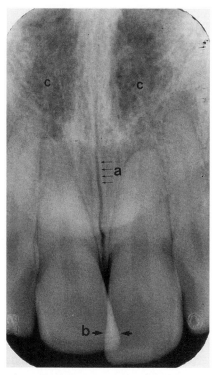

Figure 11–4. Central incisor view.

a. Intermaxillary surface (median palatine suture).

b. Overlap of enamel.

c. Nasal fossa.

Can you identify the anterior nasal spine?

Can you identify the soft tissue of the nose?

Can you identify the intermaxillary suture in Figure 11–1?

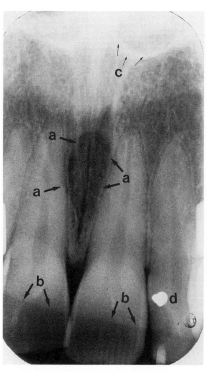

Figure 11–5. Central incisor view.

a. Incisive (nasopalatine) foramen.

b. Lip line (soft-tissue shadow of the upper lip).

c. Wall of nasal fossa.

d. Small amalgam filling in lingual pit of lateral incisor.

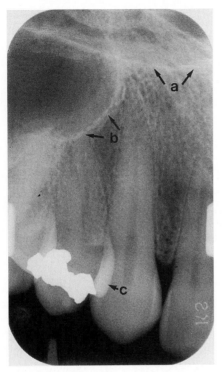

Figure 11–6. Right cuspid view.

a. Floor, or lateral wall, of nasal fossa.

b. Maxillary sinus (anterior wall). The lateral wall of the nasal fossa and the anterior wall of the maxillary sinus form an inverted "Y," called the Y line of Ennis.

c. What is that opaque (white) shadow?

Answer: The lingual cusp of the maxillary right first bicuspid premolar, usually superimposed on cuspid views.

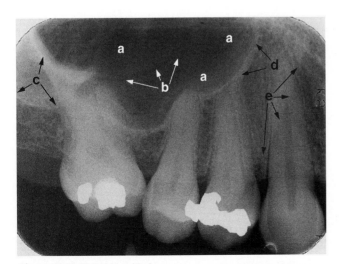

Figure 11–7. Right bicuspid view.

a. Right maxillary sinus.

b. Vascular channel (blood vessel).

c. Zygoma (cheek bone).

d. Anterior wall of maxillary sinus. (Remember, it came as far forward as the cuspid as seen in Figure 11–4).

e. Nasolabial fold (a soft-tissue shadow that runs from the ala of the nose to the corner of the lip).

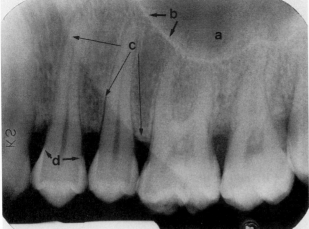

Figure 11–8. Left bicuspid view.

a. Left maxillary sinus.

b. What is this? (See Fig. 11–6, *b.*)
   Answer: The anterior wall of the maxillary sinus. It "rises" superiorly upward in the anterior (front) region.

c. What is this? (See Fig. 11–7, *e.*)

d. What is this?
   Answer: The point where enamel meets cementum, termed the CEJ, the cementoenamel junction.

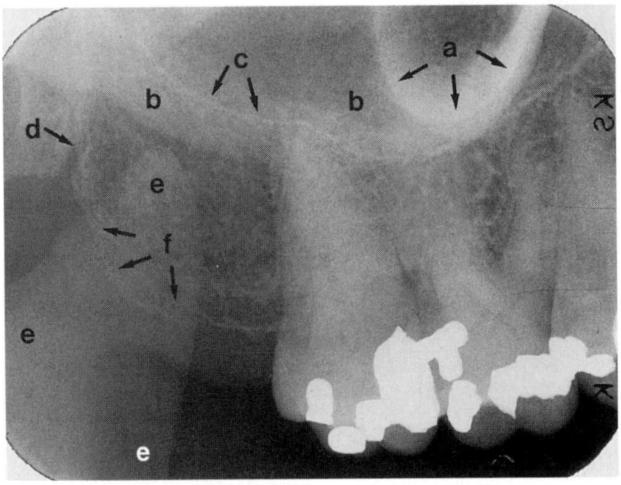

Figure 11–9. Right molar view.

a. Zygomatic process (U-shaped).

b. Body of zygomatic bone.

c. Floor of maxillary sinus (superimposed fine white line).

d. Hamular notch.

e. Coronoid process.

f. Maxillary tuberosity.

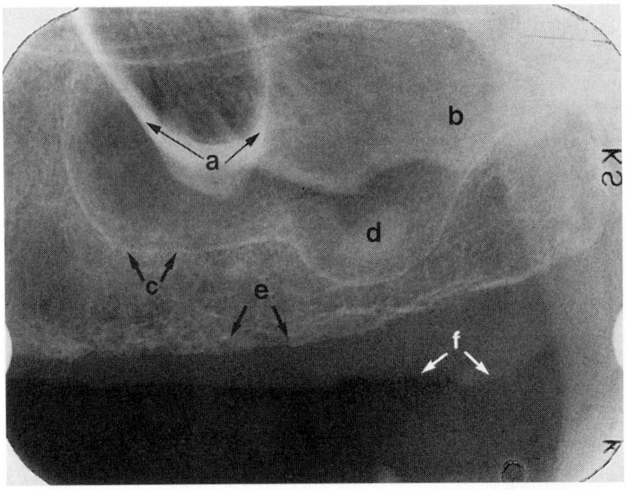

a. Zygomatic process.

b. Body of zygomatic bone.

c. Floor of maxillary sinus.

d. Root tip pushed into sinus.

e. Alveolar bone crest.

f. Soft tissue (gingiva) of ridge.

Figure 11–10. Left molar view. (Remember: the coronoid process is posterior.)

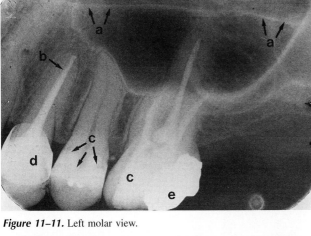

Figure 11–11. Left molar view.

a. Hard palate (also the floor of the nose).
b. Gutta-percha (root canal filling material).
c. Radiopaque (synthetic, plastic, etc.) filling.
d. Temporary metal (stainless steel) crown.
e. Amalgam (silver filling).

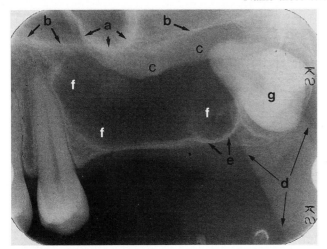

Figure 11–12. Right molar view.

a. Zygomatic process.
b. What soft-tissue structure is this? *Answer:* The hamular notch (see Fig. 11–9, *d*).
c. Hamular process—bony process of *medial* pterygoid plate.

Name these structures:

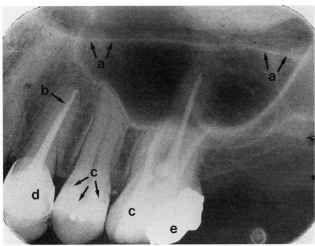

Figure 11–13. Left bicuspid view.

a. _____
(see Fig. 11–10, *a*).

b. _____
(see Fig. 11–11, *a*).

c. _____
(see Fig. 11–9, *b*).

d. _____
(see Fig. 11–9, *e*).

e. _____
(see Fig. 11–10, *c*).

f. _____
(see Fig. 11–8, *a*).

g. _____
What is this?

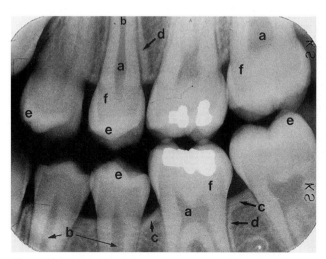

a. Pulp chamber.

b. Root chamber (pulpal canal).

c. Alveolar crest—continuous with which structure?
Answer: The lamina dura.

d. Lamina dura (surrounding entire root).

e. Enamel.

f. Dentin.

Figure 11–14. Left bitewing.

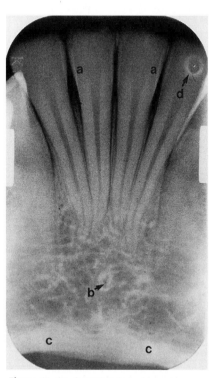

a. Mandibular central incisors.

b. Lingual foramen.

c. Inferior border of mandible.

d. Identification dot (embossed dot).

Figure 11–15. Central incisor view.

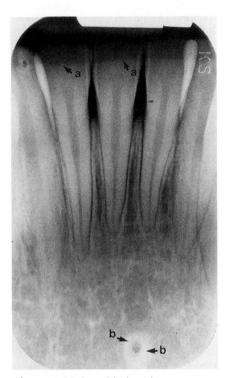

Figure 11–16. Central incisor view.

a. Lip line (soft-tissue shadow of lower lip).
b. Genial tubercles (radiopaque circle) surrounding the radiolucent lingual foramen (see Fig. 11–15).

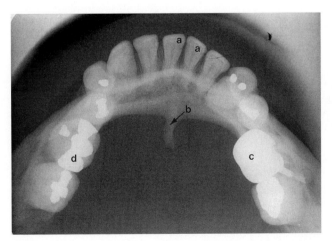

Figure 11–17. Standard occlusal view.

a. Central incisors.
b. Genial tubercles.
c. Crown.
d. Amalgam.

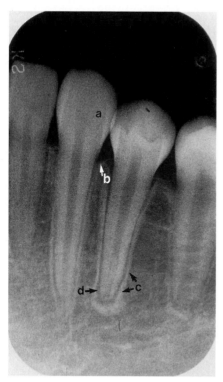

a. Mandibular left permanent cuspid.
b. Alveolar crestal bone.
c. Lamina dura.
d. Periodontal ligament space.
(This radiograph should look familiar; see Fig. 11–2.)

Figure 11–18. Left cuspid view.

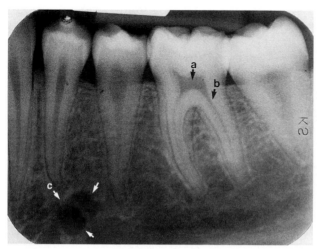

a. Pulp chamber.
b. Pulpal canal (root canal).
c. Mental foramen (almost always situated at or near bicuspid apices).

Figure 11–19. Left bicuspid view.

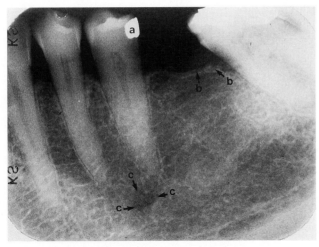

Figure 11–20. Left bicuspid view.

a. Small dental amalgam (silver filling).
b. Alveolar crest.
c. What is this structure?
   Hint: It is radiolucent (dark) and near the apices of the bicuspids (see Fig. 11–19, *c*).

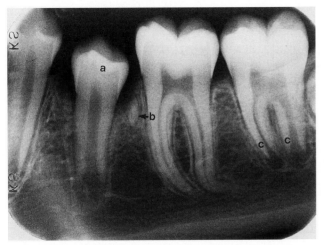

Figure 11–21. Left bicuspid view.

a. Erupting second bicuspid.
b. Retained root tip of primary molar. Which primary molar? (See Fig. 11–22.)
c. Developing apices.
   Note: The mental foramen, so prominent in Figure 11–19, is *not* visible on this film.

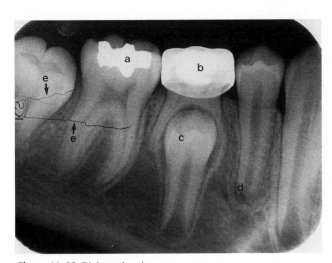

Figure 11–22. Right molar view.

a. Amalgam.
b. Stainless steel crown on second primary molar. Space maintenance is working.
c. Developing second bicuspid.
d. Developing apex of first bicuspid, which erupts at about age 9 and finishes root formation approximately 3 years later. Therefore, the patient's age is _____.
   Hint: The "12-year" molar has not quite erupted.
e. Artifact.

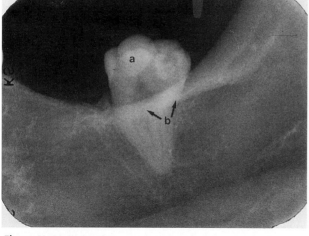

Figure 11–23. Molar view.

a. Permanent third molar (wisdom tooth).
b. External oblique ridge.

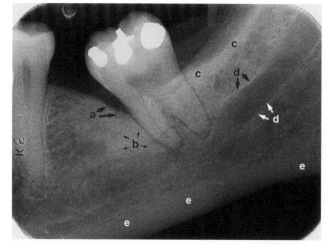

Figure 11–24. Molar view.

a. Vertical bone defect.
b. Reactive bone.
c. External oblique ridge.
d. Mandibular canal (inferior alveolar canal).
e. Lower cortical border.

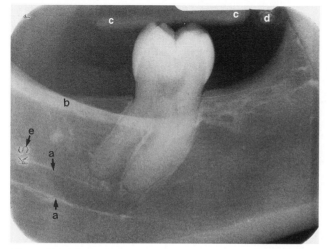

Figure 11–25. Molar view.

a. Mandibular canal.
b. External oblique ridge.
c. Plastic biteblock.
d. Identification dot.
e. Film code (manufacturer's).

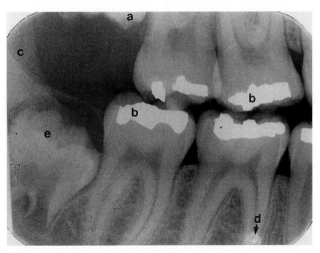

a. Developing unerupted maxillary third molar.

b. Amalgams.

c. Ascending ramus.

d. Raised dot.

e. Follicle and developing mandibular right third molar.

Figure 11–26. Right molar bitewing.

TIPS ON MOUNTING DENTAL RADIOGRAPHS

For the new student of dental radiology, the mounting of radiographs can be frustrating. Some clinicians or institutions like to have the raised (embossed) dot facing upward, and some like it downward. If the raised dot faces the observer, the patient's right side is seen on the left portion of an x-ray mount. Initially, this causes confusion for everyone—the student, the patient, and the clinician—unless a routine method of mounting is established. A catchy phrase (mnemonic) to help you remember is "It's a pimple, not a dimple." A pimple sticks out, a dimple is a depression.

Because this raised dot is always oriented toward the tubehead during exposure (so that the sensitive side of the film packet faces the x-ray source), it is reasonable to maintain this orientation when viewing the exposed film or radiograph. Thus, "right is left, and left is right," just as when you look at your patient's face: the patient's right is your left, and vice versa. If you always orient your films so that the dot is raised (Fig. 11–27), it will be easy for you to determine which part of your film is anterior and which is posterior, if you have a good knowledge of normal anatomy.

Many instructors teach their students to put the "dot in the slot" when placing the x-ray film in the holding device. By always orienting the dot toward the incisal or occlusal surface ("in the slot"), you make sure that the dot will never be superimposed over anatomic structures, and this procedure will help to correctly orient your films. This technique tip does not apply to bitewing films, because all incisal or occlusal edges are in the *middle* of the bitewing film.

Figure 11–28 illustrates both the correct orientation of the dot in a periapical view *(A)* and its possible position on a bitewing film *(B)*.

With the assumption that the embossed dot faces upward, the next section demonstrates how anatomic landmarks help you to orient films correctly.

Maxillary Films

The tooth that is centered in Figure 11–29 is a maxillary lateral incisor. Is it from the left or right side of the maxillary arch? First you must determine which side of the film is anterior and which side is posterior.

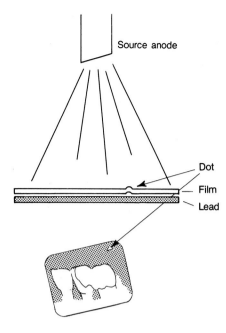

Source anode

Dot

Film

Lead

Figure 11–27. Orienting the films so that the embossed dot is raised makes it easier to determine which parts of the film are anterior and which parts are posterior. Remember, the raised dot should feel like a "pimple" not a "dimple."

Which tooth is the central incisor? It is the one to the right of the lateral incisor. Therefore, the midline, or the front (anterior) part of the mouth, is to the right side of the film.

This tooth is the maxillary *right* lateral incisor. The maxillary right cuspid is distal to the lateral incisor. (Recall that the lingual cusp, *e* in Figure 11–29, of the incisor is usually overlapped onto the distal cusp of the cuspid.)

How does the knowledge of normal anatomy confirm this conclusion? Look at the structure labeled *a* in Figure 11–29. It is the maxillary sinus. It ends near the maxillary cuspid region. Therefore, *d* must be the maxillary cuspid. It has the right shape, and its root length is appropriately longer than that of the lateral incisor. What is *b* then? It is the nasal fossa. (See Fig. 11–4, *c*.)

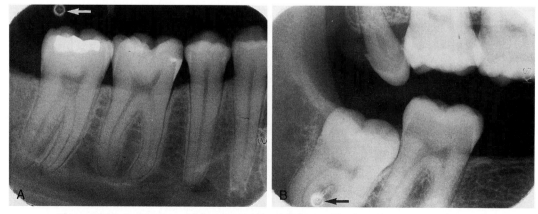

Figure 11–28. An illustration of the correct *(A)* and incorrect *(B)* orientation of the raised dot in a periapical view.

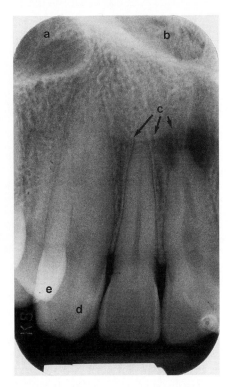

Figure 11–29. Maxillary lateral view.

The arrows pointing to structure *c* in Figure 11–29, then, demonstrate the right ala (wing) of the nose.

In Figure 11–30, structure *a* is the maxillary cuspid. What is *b*? It is the nasolabial fold. This fold always runs obliquely *downward* in an anterior (front)-to-posterior (back) direction. Therefore, this must be a maxillary left bicuspid view. How can we confirm this?

Look at the structure labeled *c*. This is the maxillary sinus. Notice that it rises in the region of the bicuspid. The section rising is the anterior wall of the

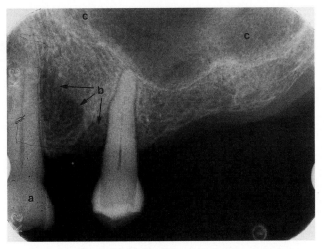

Figure 11–30. Maxillary posterior view.

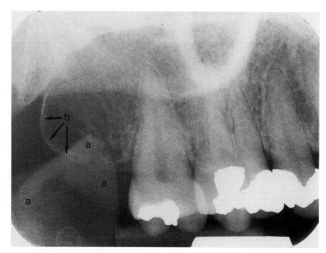

Figure 11–31. Maxillary posterior view.

maxillary sinus (see Fig. 11–6, *b*): it rises in the anterior region. With the correct identification of both the maxillary sinus and the shadow of the nasolabial fold, you can properly mount the films of edentulous or partially edentulous regions.

In Figure 11–31, what is the structure labeled *a*? It is the coronoid process. Is it anterior or posterior in the mouth? It is posterior. What is the structure labeled *b*? It is the tuberosity. It, too, is posterior. Therefore, the left side of the film is the posterior and the right side is the anterior. This must be a maxillary *right* molar view (because right is left, and vice versa).

In Figure 11–32, what is the structure labeled *a*? What is the structure labeled *b*? What is this view? (There is a catch.)

The maxillary first bicuspid has been extracted. The operator here decided to use one film to record all the teeth from the cuspid to the second molar. Therefore, this is a premolar view that records all the posterior teeth. This view was possible only because the operator knew that both the first bicuspid and the third molar

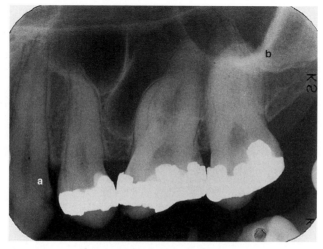

Figure 11–32. Maxillary posterior view.

had been previously extracted. The structure *a* is a cuspid; *b* is the zygomatic process. Can you identify the hard palate (floor of the nasal cavity)?

Mandibular Films

The mandibular central incisor view (Fig. 11–33) should not be difficult to identify. As long as the dot *(arrow)* is raised, you can identify

- *a* as the mandibular *right* central incisor.
- *b* as the mandibular *right* lateral incisor.
- *c* as the mandibular *left* central incisor.

Is Figure 11–34 a maxillary or a mandibular cuspid view? What anatomic space, or lucency, is seen in a maxillary cuspid view? The sinus. Is it seen here? No. What is the structure labeled *a* (see Fig. 11–25)? It is *mandibular* cortical bone. Therefore, because the film shows no sinus, but it does show a view of the mandibular cortex, this must be a *mandibular* view, in which

- *b* is the mandibular central incisor.
- *c* is the mandibular lateral incisor.
- *d* is the first bicuspid.

We can conclude that this is the mandibular *left* cuspid view.

Figure 11–35 is a molar view. Can you identify the structure labeled *a*? It is the external oblique ridge (see Figs. 11–24 and 11–25) and is in the posterior part of the mouth. Therefore, this is a mandibular left molar view. The anterior part of

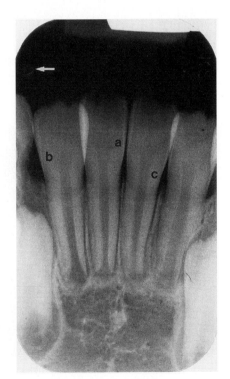

Figure 11–33. Mandibular central incisor view.

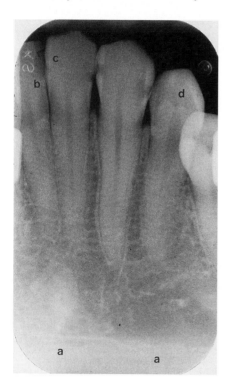

Figure 11–34. Cuspid view.

the mouth is to your left. The external oblique ridge always runs obliquely downward from posterior to anterior.

Summary

These illustrations demonstrate that you must always rely on your knowledge of normal anatomy to mount the radiographs that you expose. Remember that the embossed dot should always be raised. "It's a *pimple*, not a dimple." You can feel

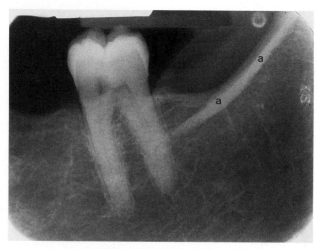

Figure 11–35. Molar view.

the "bump" of the dot with your fingers. An incorrectly mounted radiograph could result in the wrong dental procedure being performed.

Review this chapter until you feel confident that you can identify the normal anatomic landmarks accurately. Refer to this chapter if you have any doubts about the correct orientation of any films.

MOUNTING PROCEDURE

Step 1. Collect the *dry* films, and sit at a view box in a quiet atmosphere with a prepared mount. Place the films on a light-colored surface (not the view box). Many viewing areas have black countertops, which are good for viewing but sometimes make it difficult to see where the films are lying on the countertop. If this is the case, place the films on a piece of white paper.

Step 2. Turn all of the films so that the embossed dot is raised (toward you). The American Dental Association recommends that radiographs be mounted and viewed from the facial aspect—that is, from the outside inward. While standing in front of the patient, if you hold the mounted set of films next to the patient's head, the structures in the films will match the structures in the patient's mouth. The films of the right side of the patient's mouth will be on the patient's right side (your left). Think of looking at the films as if you were looking at the patient.

Step 3. Group all of the maxillary films together, all of the mandibular films together, and all of the bitewing films together (use the "Helpful Hints" provided later in this chapter). Then turn the films so that all of the occlusal surfaces and the incisal edges in the maxillary films point downward and the occlusal surfaces and the incisal edges of the mandibular films point upward (just as they grow in the mouth). Set the bitewing views aside temporarily.

Step 4. After you think you have placed the films in the correct order, insert them into the corresponding frames of the mount.

Step 5. Place the bitewing films on the appropriate side between the maxillary posterior periapical views and the mandibular posterior periapical views.

Step 6. *Final check*: Looking at the back of the mount, check to see that the dots are all in the same location. At the front of the mount, the patient's name and the exposure date should be plainly visible, and the overall curve of the occlusal/incisal edges should make the survey look as if it is smiling.

Helpful Hints for Anatomic Landmark Identification in Intraoral Radiographs

1. The teeth are oriented with the longer side of the film vertical for anterior teeth and horizontal for posterior teeth.
2. Mandibular anterior teeth have smaller crowns and shorter roots than do maxillary anterior teeth.
3. The four mandibular incisors usually fit on one film, whereas the four maxillary incisors, being larger, may not.
4. The maxillary central incisor film shows the median palatine suture, which creates a distinct radiolucent line between the maxillary incisors that is not present between the mandibular incisors (see Fig. 11–2).
5. Mandibular molars normally have only two roots, the image of which is

very sharp and distinct. Maxillary molars have three roots, the image of which is less distinct than that of the mandibular teeth.

6. The direction of curvature is distal for most normally curving roots.

7. Maxillary radiographs have larger radiolucent areas: the nasal fossa in the anterior region and the maxillary sinuses in the posterior region of the apices. These radiolucent areas would not appear in mandibular films.

8. The posterior border of the maxilla has an area called the *tuberosity* that looks like a rounded corner (see Fig. 11–6).

9. Some teeth may have restorations that will help you to determine what is imaged on the films.

10. The overall appearance of a complete mouth radiographic survey (CMRS) or bitewing (BW) survey presents the occlusal plane in an upward curve that looks like a smile from the anterior to the posterior sides.

Study Questions

1. Which of the following structures is considered to be radiolucent?
   A. Anterior nasal spine.
   B. Zygomatic process.
   C. Intermaxillary or medial palatine suture.
   D. Lamina dura.

2. Which of the following structures is considered to be radiopaque?
   A. Incisive foramen.
   B. Periodontal ligament.
   C. Maxillary sinus.
   D. Genial tubercles.

3. When you view mounted radiographs, it is recommended that the raised dot be facing toward you. This helps you orient the structures on the film. Which of the following statements is true about your orientation of the film?
   A. The patient's left is on your left.
   B. You are looking at the patient's teeth as if you were sitting on the patient's tongue looking out.
   C. The patient's right is on your left.
   D. You cannot tell which is the patient's right or left unless the films are labeled.

4. Which of the following is not a helpful hint for mounting radiographs?
   A. Mandibular teeth usually have smaller crowns and shorter roots than maxillary teeth.
   B. The longer side of the film is usually vertical for posterior teeth and horizontal for anterior teeth.
   C. Maxillary molars usually have three roots, and mandibular molars usually have two roots.
   D. The overall appearance of the radiographic survey will have an upward curve like a smile.

5. Have you answered the questions that appear next to Figure 11–13?

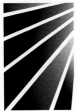

Chapter 12

Interpretation: Normal Versus Abnormal and Common Radiographic Presentation of Lesions

DETECTION OF DISEASE

Diagnoses are not made from radiographs alone; the radiograph is only one tool. For many disorders, such as dental caries, periodontal disease, or trauma, the radiograph is a *sensitive* detector—it shows changes in the patient's mouth. With these disorders, it is also quite *specific*—the radiographic features are specific to certain conditions. In other disorders, such as periapical infection or dental cysts and tumors, although one can detect the disease by means of radiography, one cannot precisely name the specific tumor or cyst by studying the radiographic features alone. With these disorders, the radiograph is *less specific*. Nevertheless, the intraoral radiograph is an indispensable diagnostic tool when properly used.

Dental auxiliaries can play a significant role in disease detection. As a dental team member, the well-trained auxiliary should be able to differentiate abnormal from normal radiographic features. Armed with a sound knowledge of normal anatomy, the dental assistant or dental hygienist becomes an additional detector of disease processes in the patient. In this way, the quality of the patient's care is enhanced.

This chapter illustrates radiographic features of common dental diseases and anomalies that may be visualized on intraoral radiographs. In a comparative approach, examples of abnormal processes are illustrated together with normal anatomic structures. For purposes of comparison, the following categories of radiographic changes are used:

1. Radiographic changes owing to **trauma**.
2. Radiographic changes owing to **periapical infection**.
3. Radiographic changes owing to **periodontal disease**.
4. Radiographic changes owing to **dental caries**.
5. Radiographic features of **dental anomalies**.

BASIC VIEWING PRINCIPLES

Detecting differences between normal and abnormal structures involves more than just a casual glance at the films. Certain viewing strategies maximize the information garnered from a set of radiographs.

Viewing Conditions

1. You must begin with *good* films—properly placed, exposed, processed, and mounted.

2. The viewing area should be quiet, be free of distractions, and have subdued lighting.
3. You should have a magnifying glass.
4. You should look at multiple film views, if available.

Viewing Technique

Keep these basic factors in mind as you view the films:

1. Follow a consistent pattern. For example:
   a. Start left to right, viewing maxillary films first.
   b. Take an overview of the patient's set of films. Stand back and look at the set as a whole.
   c. Begin surveying the supporting structures of the teeth, then follow the outline of the roots and the crowns.
   d. Finally, move your gaze inward to the internal structure of the teeth.
2. Use constant eye movement. Do not stare at the films. The differences in shades of gray will fade as you stare.
3. Watch for possible indicators of abnormality, such as
   a. *Breaks in continuity.* Does the lamina dura have a break in it, or is there a dark spot in the white outline of the enamel?
   b. *Asymmetry.* Are there obvious differences from one side of the patient to the other when you see a radiolucency or radiopacity? Is there also one on the other side?
   c. *Change in size.* Are there any dimensional changes, expansion of the bone, or changes in shape of the teeth or jaws?

Radiographic Interpretation

This chapter is not an exhaustive review of oral pathology or radiographic interpretation. It is designed to sensitize the dental auxiliary student to common dental abnormalities. We hope that by comparing normal and abnormal structures, you will reinforce your knowledge of normal radiographic anatomic landmarks and will become proficient at detecting abnormal features that might affect patient care.

At the end of this chapter, a series of line drawings outline typical radiographic presentations of pathologic lesions. These diagrams are followed by multiple radiographic examples of odontogenic cysts and tumors to compare against the line drawings. A discussion of the etiology, clinical characteristics, and histologic features of these lesions is beyond the scope of this textbook. The reader is directed to another of our textbooks for this information.*

RADIOGRAPHIC CHANGES RESULTING FROM TRAUMA

Discussion. The radiolucent (dark) structure labeled *a* in Figure 12–1 is the incisive foramen. It is a normal anatomic landmark seen between the roots of the

---

*Miles D, VanDis M, Kaugars G, Lovas J. Oral and Maxillofacial Radiology, Radiologic/Pathologic Correlations, Philadelphia, WB Saunders, 1991.

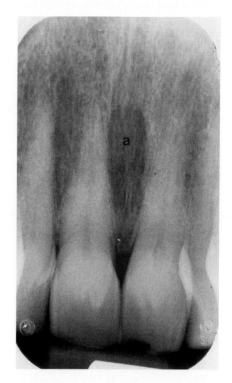

Figure 12–1. Incisive foramen *(a)*.

maxillary central incisors. Clinically, one would see a "bump" (the incisive papilla) on the palate directly behind the central incisors. The foramen lies below this bump.

By comparison, *b* in Figure 12–2 is *not* situated between the roots of the central incisors. This radiolucency is located periapically; that is, it lies at the root end of the tooth. It is also more hydraulic (round) than *a* in this radiograph, and it is *large*. The area labeled *c* in Figure 12–2 is an incisive fracture. Thus, one may surmise that the area has probably sustained trauma. The right maxillary incisor was fractured. Pulp tissue in the left incisor died, with subsequent abscess and local bone destruction at the apex of the tooth.

Summary. We know that object *b* in Figure 12–2 is *not* the incisive foramen because of

1. Its location (periapical).
2. Its size (large).
3. Its shape (the foramen is most often oval or heart-shaped).
4. The evidence of previous trauma to the region.

Discussion. Children as well as adults often sustain trauma to their teeth. The pulp may degenerate or die, producing an apical lesion such as the one seen in Figure 12–2. Another consequence of trauma may be total atrophy of the pulp, with a calcified pulp canal, as seen in tooth no. 51 (the right primary central incisor) in Figure 12–3. This tooth must be watched by the clinician, as an infection might later result from this compromised tooth and could affect the developing tooth *a* in this figure.

Discussion. In Figure 12–4, *a* is a fracture line that followed a blow to the maxillary incisors, as is *c*. A similar line, labeled *b*, crosses several teeth in both

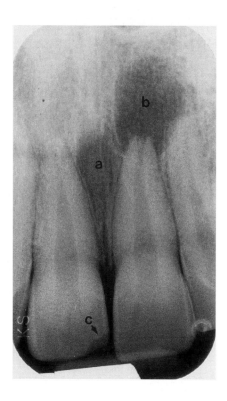

Figure 12–2. Incisive foramen *(a)*; apical lesion (the periapical radiolucency), probably a radicular cyst *(b)*; and incisal fracture *(c)*.

Figure 12–3. Tooth no. 51 shows no radiographic evidence of a pulp chamber or canal. Compare this tooth with the left primary central incisor, no. 61, which has a pulp chamber *(p)*.

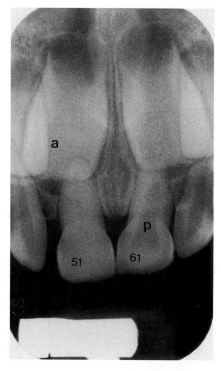

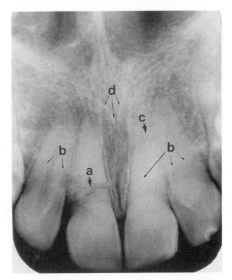

Figure 12–4. Fracture in tooth no. 11 *(a)*, shadow of the nose *(b)*, fracture in tooth no. 21 *(c)*, and anterior nasal spine *(d)*.

Figure 12–4 and Figure 12–5. This line, however, represents the outline of the soft tissue of the nose. Whereas the outline of the nose is a smooth line, fracture lines are usually jagged or interrupted.

Question. Which apex do you think is abnormal, *a* in Figure 12–6 or *a* in Figure 12–7?

Discussion. Another consequence of trauma to a tooth can be external resorption (the erosion or destruction of the root end). Figure 12–6 shows a central incisor with an "open" apex and a wide pulp chamber. Figure 12–7 shows a similar situation. Whereas the apex of the lateral incisor in Figure 12–6 is closed, all the apices of the incisors in Figure 12–7 are open. The root of the central incisor in Figure 12–6 failed to develop because of injury. Its pulp chamber remained large, unlike the normal-appearing pulp chamber of the lateral incisor. The pulp chambers and apices of the four incisors in Figure 12–7 are normal and are still undergoing development.

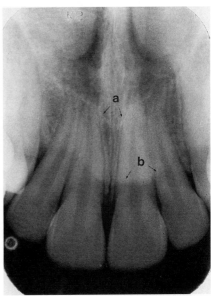

Figure 12–5. Anterior nasal spine *(a)* and shadow of the nose *(b)*.

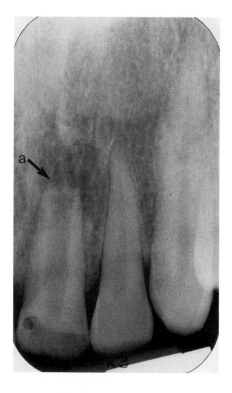

Figure 12–6. Apex of left central incisor *(a)*.

RADIOGRAPHIC CHANGES RESULTING FROM PERIAPICAL INFECTION

The most common radiographic appearance of a periapical infection is the *periapical radiolucency*—a "black hole" at the apex of a tooth. The origin of these black holes may be pulpal or periodontal; an area of bone destruction results from the death of the pulp as a consequence of deep decay (pulpal origin) or as an

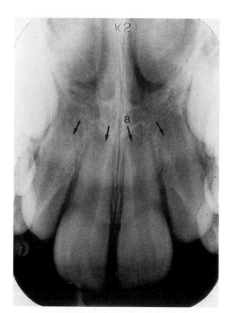

Figure 12–7. Apex of left central incisor *(a)*.

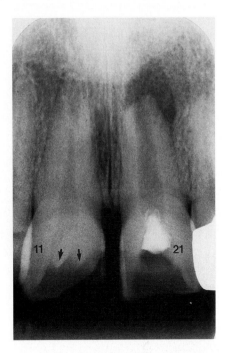

Figure 12–8. Pulp death of tooth no. 21 probably resulted from a carious lesion in the developmental pit area on the lingual aspect of the tooth. Note the talons (or extra cusps) on tooth no. 11 *(arrows)*. Endodontic treatment has been started on the periapically involved tooth.

extension of a periodontal bone defect that involves the apical region secondarily (periodontal origin).

Figures 12–8 through 12–11 show various radiographic appearances of dental periapical radiolucencies produced by deep carious lesions.

Discussion. After examining these typical examples of periapical radiolucencies,

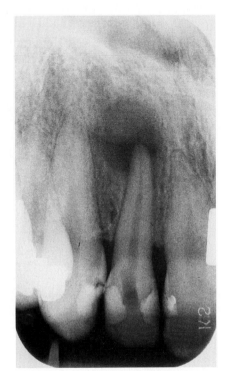

Figure 12–9. Restored carious lesions on several anterior teeth. The pulp death and apical problem could have resulted from either the initial decay or the recurrent decay seen around the restorations.

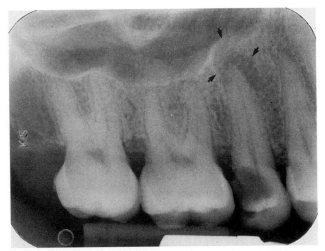

Figure 12–10. Periapical radiolucency *(arrows)* approaching the floor of the maxillary sinus.

one sees that the only normal anatomic structures in the jaws that could mimic a periapical radiolucency are

1. The incisive foramen (see Fig. 12–1).
2. The mental foramen (Fig. 12–11).

The mental foramen is labeled *mf* in Figure 12–11. This tooth has neither a cavity nor periodontal involvement. Consequently, there is no reason for the black hole to be pathologic. In contrast, the area at the apex of the first molar, labeled *a*, shows widened periodontal ligament space, proliferation of reactive bone (shown by *arrows*), and a deep cavity "temporized" by a *zinc oxide and eugenol* (ZOE) base.

Periodontal involvement of the apex of a tooth is usually by direct extension of inflammation in cases of advanced periodontitis with deep bony defects. Figures 12–12 and 12–13 show examples of this type of periapical involvement.

These defects should be easily recognized on intraoral radiographs.

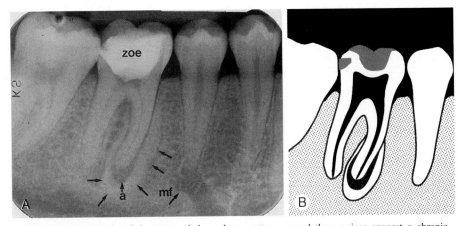

Figure 12–11. Apical radiolucency and dense bone pattern around these apices suggest a chronic, long-standing pulpal infection that the host's defenses tried to "wall off." The temporary pulp-capping procedure has failed. The structure labeled *mf* is the mental foramen (recall Chapter 11); *a* is the widened periodontal ligament space; *zoe* is the zinc oxide and eugenol base; and *arrows* indicate the proliferation of reactive bone.

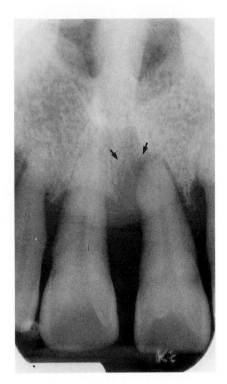

Figure 12–12. Advanced periodontal bone loss with direct extension to the apex of tooth no. 9. *Arrows* indicate the greatest vertical defect.

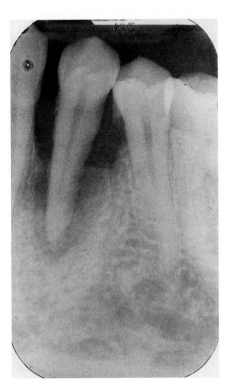

Figure 12–13. Periapical radiolucency of periodontal origin. Note the large deposits of calculus (see also Fig. 12–14).

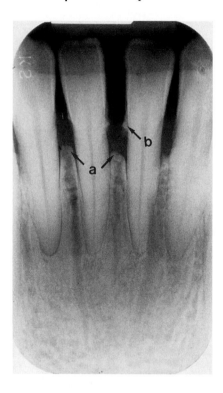

Figure 12–14. Mild blunting of crestal bone *(a)* and calculus *(b).*

RADIOGRAPHIC CHANGES RESULTING FROM PERIODONTAL DISEASE

Discussion. Minimal bone loss is seen in *a* in Figure 12–14, but the calculus "spurs," or deposits, seen in *b* suggest local factors for periodontitis. More severe bone loss and *more calculus* are seen in Figure 12–15.

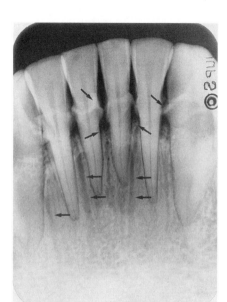

Figure 12–15. Calculus deposits in the mandibular central incisor region *(arrows).*

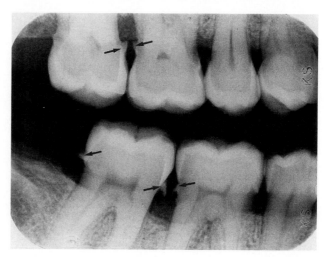

Figure 12–16. Example of calculus deposits *(arrows)* in the posterior dentition in both the mandible and the maxilla.

Figure 12–15 reveals calculus spurs in their most common location: the mandibular central incisor region. Note the horizontal bone loss. Note also the multiple vertical radiolucent lines. These vascular channels are sometimes referred to as *nutrient canals* (seen also in Fig. 12–14). They are another sign of chronic inflammatory change associated with periodontal disease. Figure 12–16 is a good example of calculus deposits in the posterior dentition, both in the mandible and in the maxilla. No cavities are present here (the chapter gives examples of cavities later), and as yet there is little bone loss.

Figure 12–17 reveals *advanced*, localized bone loss in the posterior maxilla. Note that the bony defect is primarily in the second bicuspid region.

Discussion. Periodontal disease, when active and chronic, will lead to advanced bone loss if untreated. Local factors such as plaque and calculus, in the presence of inflammation, complicate the injury. Chronic inflammation, toxins, and enzymes cause breakdown of the periodontium (gingiva and bone). The ravages of these

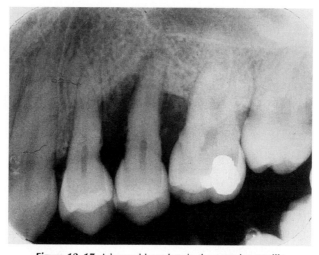

Figure 12–17. Advanced bone loss in the posterior maxilla.

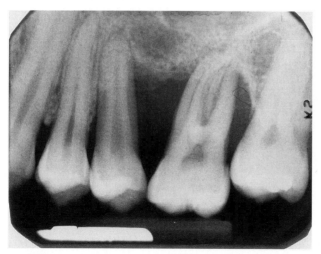

Figure 12–18. Bone loss resulting from juvenile periodontitis.

processes are reflected radiographically by bone loss and other defects. Both horizontal bone loss and vertical bone defects may be present. The radiographic changes may be localized to one area or generalized throughout the dentition. But the radiographic picture reflects only the changes that have occurred, not whether the process is *currently* active. Periodontitis with associated bone change is a recurring disease with periods of inactivity or remission. Other factors besides plaque and calculus may affect the nature of the bone involvement.

Systemic diseases such as diabetes or other immunologic problems may impair the patient's ability to mount a defense against infection. Classification and discussion of the various types of periodontal diseases are available in other dental textbooks and are beyond the scope of this text. Suffice it to say, when severe periodontal bone loss is localized to the first molar and central incisor regions, or when the severity of the disease is not proportional to the local factors present, a search should be made for a systemic cause for the bone loss. Figures 12–18 and 12–19 show bone loss in a 20-year-old woman with juvenile periodontitis, one

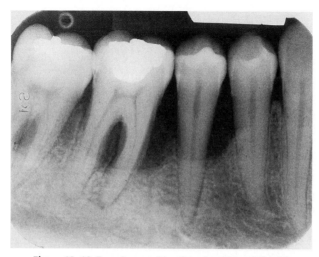

Figure 12–19. Bone loss resulting from juvenile periodontitis.

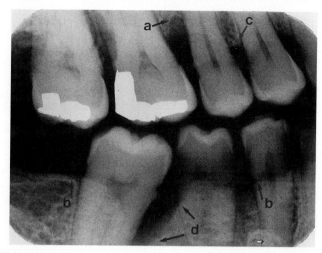

Figure 12–20. Vertical bone defect *(a)*, crestal ridge at near-normal height *(b)*, alveolar crest *(c)*, and severe vertical defect *(d)*.

type of severe periodontal disease. Note the bone changes in these films, and compare the location of the defects with those in the localized severe periodontitis pictured in Figure 12–20.

Discussion. Localized severe periodontal bone defects appear as sharp, angular bone margins. In contrast, healthy alveolar bone has an intact crestal margin (Fig. 12–21) and is radiographically visible about 1 mm to 2 mm apical to the cementoenamel junction (CEJ).

Discussion. In the maxillary or mandibular anterior region, the picture is different. Figure 12–22 illustrates the alveolar crestal bone as sharp points or crests between each incisor in a healthy individual. By contrast, the bone level *b* in Figure 12–23 represents the typical picture of the ''blunting'' of the alveolar crests as a result of chronic periodontitis. Note also the presence of vascular channels and calculus spurs, which supports the diagnosis of periodontitis.

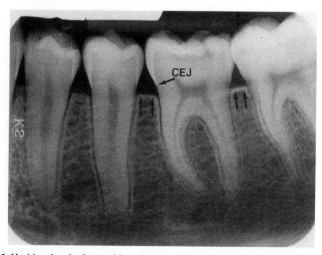

Figure 12–21. Healthy alveolar bone with an intact crestal margin; *CEJ* is the cementoenamel junction.

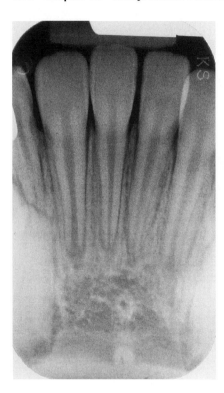

Figure 12–22. Healthy interdental, or septal, bone in mandibular anterior region.

Figure 12–23. Blunting of the alveolar crests *(b)* as a result of chronic periodontitis. *Upper arrows* show calculus deposits; *lower arrows* show nutrient canals.

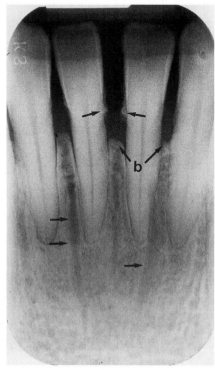

RADIOGRAPHIC CHANGES RESULTING FROM DENTAL CARIES

The dental auxiliary is often the first person to view the films after they are processed. If carious lesions are detected as the films are mounted, they can be pointed out to the dentist. The dentist holds the ultimate responsibility for caries detection—the dentist decides what to treat—but the dental auxiliary should help with caries detection.

Where to Look for Dental Caries

Dental carious lesions that occur interproximally (between the teeth) are best detected on bitewing radiographs. The point of the carious attack on this part of the tooth is at or just apical to the contact point. Figure 12–24 shows the typical

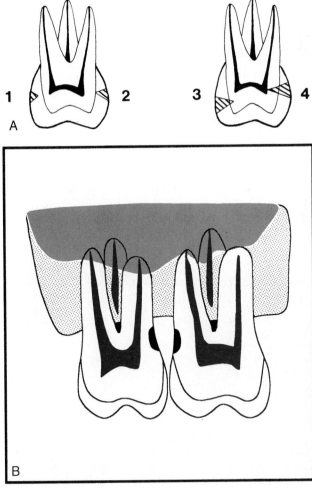

Figure 12–24. A, Typical radiographic classes of interproximal carious lesions. *B,* Root caries apical to cementoenamel junction as a result of bone loss and different locations of bacteria and food debris. Lesions are usually rounded and somewhat indistinct.

radiographic classes of interproximal carious lesions. Figure 12–24B illustrates root surface caries interproximally. Note that the lesions are well apical to the contact point owing to periodontal bone loss.

Radiographic Classification of Caries

1. **Class I caries**: Less than halfway into the enamel.
2. **Class II caries**: More than halfway into the enamel.
3. **Class III caries**: Involving the detinoenamel junction, but less than half the distance to the pulp chamber.
4. **Class IV caries**: More than half the distance to the pulp chamber.
5. **Class V caries**: Root surface caries.

Compare the illustrated carious lesions in Figure 12–24 with the actual dental caries in Figure 12–25. Figure 12–25 is a molar view of a young patient (7–8 years old) that demonstrates at least two classes of interproximal carious lesions:

a. Mandibular first primary molar, Class II, distal.
b. Mandibular second primary molar, Class II, mesial and distal.
c. Maxillary second primary molar, Class II, distal.
d. Maxillary first primary molar, Class IV (large), distal.

All of the cavities in Figure 12–25 involved the dentinoenamel junction (DEJ). The cavity on the maxillary first primary molar *(d)* has destroyed much of the back half of the tooth. It has almost reached the pulp chamber. Luckily for this youngster, the primary molar is about to exfoliate (be shed) as the first permanent premolar *(p)* erupts.

A classic interproximal carious lesion appears on the distal surface of the mandibular right second premolar in Figure 12–26. It is a triangular defect, with its point toward the dentin. It has not yet reached the DEJ, but it is more than halfway into the enamel. It is therefore a Class II carious lesion.

A similar lesion is seen on the tooth's mesial surface; however, its shape is less

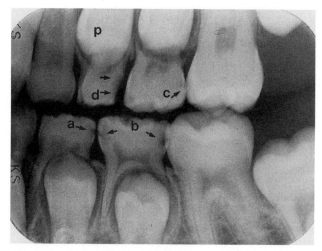

Figure 12–25. Two types of carious lesions: Class II lesions appear on teeth nos. 65 *(c)*, 74 *(a)*, and 75 *(b)*; a Class IV lesion is seen on tooth no. 64 *(d)*.

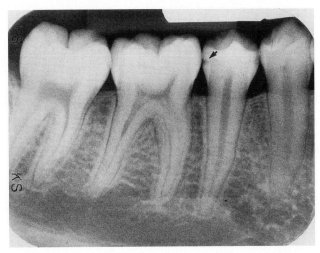

Figure 12–26. Classic interproximal carious lesion *(arrow)* on the distal surface of the mandibular right second premolar.

pronounced. Some interproximal cavities are less conspicuous because of variance in enamel thickness, thickness of the patient's hard and soft tissues, overlying soft tissue, degree of enamel destruction, or variable technique factors. Cavities of all types, marked with arrows, appear in Figure 12–27. Note how much less conspicuous are the lesions on the second premolar and second molar than is the large cavity on the first molar.

On what surface of the second molar is the cavity marked *a* in Figure 12–28 (seen here as a circular radiolucency)? It may be either buccal (facial) or lingual. Remember that a radiograph is a two-dimensional "picture."

One cannot tell from the x-ray film alone which side—the buccal or the lingual—the cavity is located on. This fact must be confirmed clinically.

Cavities may spread along the junction of dentin and enamel in a linear fashion, whether they are interproximal or occlusal cavities. An occlusal cavity is one that

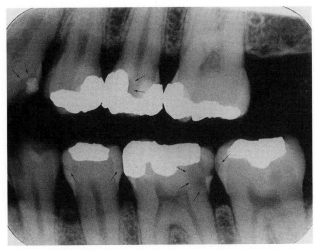

Figure 12–27. Carious lesions: tooth no. 23, distal, recurrent; tooth no. 25, mesial, recurrent; tooth no. 35, mesial and distal, Class I or II; tooth no. 36, distal, Class IV; and tooth no. 37, mesial, Class I.

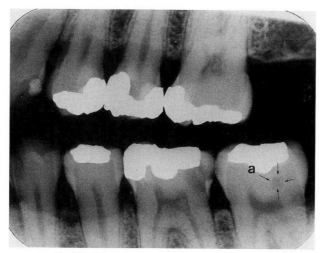

Figure 12–28. Facial *(buccal)* or lingual caries *(a).* This is the same radiograph as Figure 12–27. Find the same lesion on Figure 12–28 without the arrows to guide you.

starts on the biting surface of a posterior tooth in the developmental pit and fissure areas. In Figure 12–29, the letter *a* shows the radiographic appearance of a typical occlusal cavity. An earlier, more subtle occlusal cavity is seen at the DEJ on the second molar as a radiolucent line marked *b.*

Cavities may also recur, or begin anew, under margins of existing fillings (restorations). In Figure 12–30, we see two examples of rather large carious lesions, both interproximal, that appear around or beneath existing amalgam restorations.

Dental caries, if left untreated, can destroy large amounts of the tooth. Figure 12–31 reveals one side of a patient's mouth, where many advanced carious lesions are visible radiographically. Only root "stumps" are left of the maxillary premolars and the second molar. Similarly, only root tips remain of the mandibular first molar.

This type of rampant dental decay is not limited to adults. Figure 12–32 is the

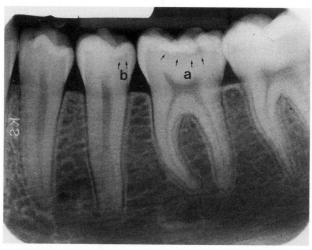

Figure 12–29. Carious lesions *(a)* that have begun on the occlusal surface. The cavity marked *b* began in the distal pit of this bicuspid.

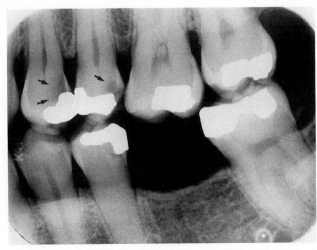

Figure 12–30. Two examples of large interproximal carious lesions *(arrows)* around or beneath existing amalgam restorations.

bitewing radiograph of an 8-year-old boy with a gross carious lesion on the maxillary first primary molar (see arrows). The maxillary second primary molar has been restored conservatively with silver amalgam. The mandibular primary molars have had pulpotomies (removal of the pulp tissue), and "temporary" stainless steel crowns had been placed on the primary molars. The stainless steel crown on the second primary molar had fallen off; the radiograph was taken to determine why. The dark, or radiolucent, area beneath the crown of the tooth and between the roots is a large area of bone destruction caused by dental abscess. Recall the similar appearance of infection in Figures 12–10 and 12–11.

The final type of common dental caries is the cervical lesion (root cavity). Root carious lesions occur apical to the CEJ. Usually they are preceded by periodontal bone destruction of alveolar crestal bone (horizontal bone loss), with resulting exposure of the root surface in the oral cavity.

With this lower level of bone, food impaction occurs more apically on the tooth,

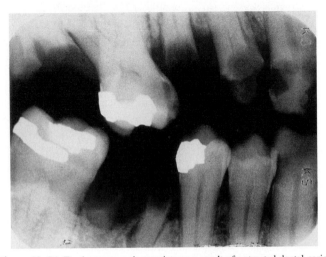

Figure 12–31. Tooth structure destruction as a result of untreated dental caries.

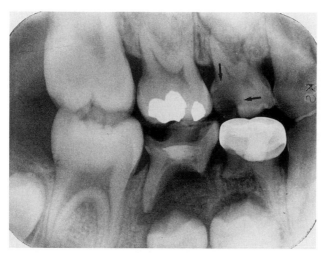

Figure 12–32. The bitewing radiograph of an 8-year-old boy with gross carious lesions on the maxillary first primary molar *(arrows).*

not just below the contact point. The plaque and bacteria accumulate in this region and lead to cervical or root decay. The radiographic appearance of root caries is different from classic interproximal decay. The cavities are *not usually triangular, but appear rounded, or cupped out.* Early lesions may be difficult to distinguish on x rays. However, if suspect radiolucencies are apical to the CEJ in the presence of horizontal bone loss, the suspicion of a root cavity should be high. A typical lesion appears in Figure 12–33 on the maxillary second premolar *a*. A less distinct lesion is seen on the molar *b*. Figure 12–34 shows a well-advanced lesion that is encroaching on the pulp. The maxillary canine (cuspid) in this radiograph most likely has a compromised pulpal vitality.

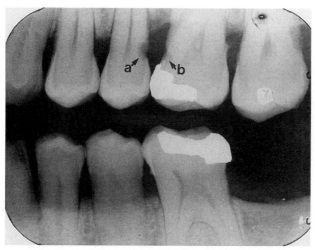

Figure 12–33. Typical lesion *(a)* on the patient's maxillary second premolar and a less distinct lesion *(b)* on the molar.

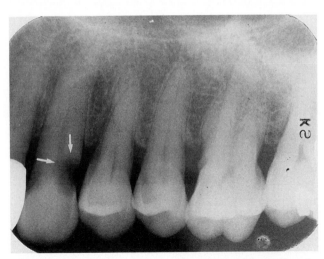

Figure 12–34. Well advanced lesion *(arrows)* encroaching on the pulp.

RADIOGRAPHIC FEATURES OF DENTAL ANOMALIES

A Potpourri of Developmental Abnormalities

Figures 12–35 and 12–36 reveal dense but diffuse radiopacities (white regions) in the mandible. They often appear bilaterally, not, that is, on both sides of the

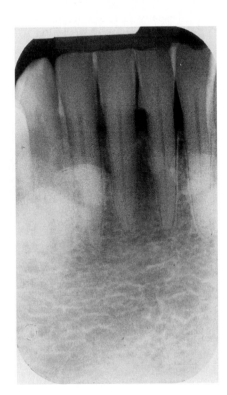

Figure 12–35. Radiopacities in the mandible.

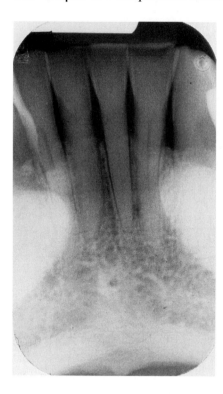

Figure 12–36. Radiopacities in the mandible.

mandible. Most structures that occur bilaterally are normal. These opacities are mandibular tori; *tori* are dense bony outgrowths of various shapes and sizes found commonly in the mandibular lingual anterior region (Fig. 12–37). In the palate, a torus is usually seen as a single, bony, hard, midline elevation (Fig. 12–38).

The small toothlike structure labeled *a* in Figure 12–39 is a *mesiodens*, which is a supernumerary (extra) "tooth" or dental structure *(dens)* that occurs in the midline area *(mesio)*. These anomalies are usually conical and are often oriented upward. If you look closely at Figure 12–39, you can detect material of enamel density at the top, or superior aspect, of the "tooth" in both views. The lesion also has a radiolucent rim, or border, which appears similar to a normal tooth follicle.

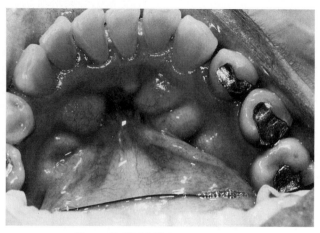

Figure 12–37. Multiple mandibular tori.

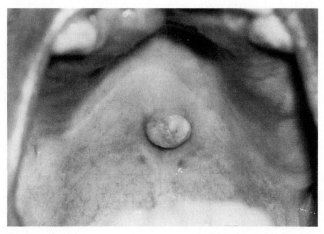

Figure 12–38. Small palatal torus. Tori can become very large over time in some patients and may interfere with film placement.

These two examples are good illustrations of the *buccal object rule* (Clark's rule, SLOB rule) discussed in Chapter 6. If the tubehead is shifted distally for the second view, and the object moves mesially—that is, in the opposite direction—then the object is on the buccal side (closer to you). Conversely, if the tubehead is shifted distally in the second film, and the object moves in the same

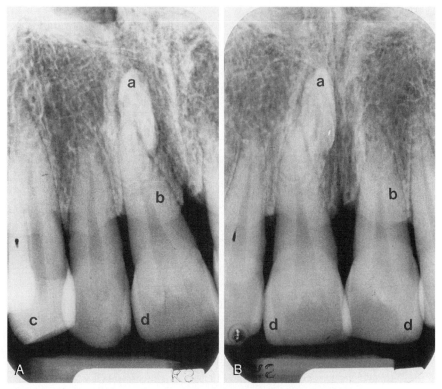

Figure 12–39. Mesiodens *(a)*, alveolar bone level *(b)*, maxillary right cuspid *(c)*, and central incisors *(d)*.

direction, then the object is on the lingual (or palatal) side. A good mnemonic device for this concept is the "SLOB rule": *S*ame on *L*ingual, *O*pposite on *B*uccal.

In this case the mesiodens is on the lingual side. Note how, as we shift from a central incisor view (mesial) to a lateral incisor view (distal), the mesiodens appears to move from a position to the right of the tooth apex in the central view to a position overlapping most of the apex in the lateral incisor view. As we move distally, it does also. Because the rule is "same on lingual, opposite on buccal," the mesiodens must be on the lingual side.

Extra dental structures besides the mesiodens also occur in the jaws. Extra teeth are called *supernumerary teeth*, as mentioned earlier. The condition of having these extra teeth is called *hyperdontia*. Hyperdontia most commonly occurs in regard to the third molar, the lateral incisor, and the premolar regions. Just as in the clinical examination, you should learn to count the teeth present on radiographs and identify which teeth are present and which are absent. One way to count teeth is to begin with an easily identifiable tooth, such as a maxillary central incisor, and then count and identify each tooth in the next most posterior view. Recall that we did this in Chapter 11 in the section on mounting. Figure 12–40 shows the radiographic appearance of an extra premolar in the right mandible. Figure 12–41 shows a maxillary supernumerary premolar that has erupted palatally in the arch. Figure 12–42 illustrates a mesiodens, a special type of supernumerary tooth, described previously.

Figure 12–43 shows an example of a "fourth" molar in the right maxilla. It has prevented the eruption of a normal-appearing third molar (wisdom tooth). Supernumerary third molars are sometimes termed *paramolars*. Smaller toothlike dental structures in this region are called *distodens*.

Figure 12–44 is a rare example of *bilateral* supernumerary lateral incisors. These incisors are so symmetrical and well formed that it is easy to miss them clinically.

Just as hyperdontia (too many teeth) is possible, so is *hypodontia* (too few teeth). Usually, there is a familial, or genetic, component to these conditions; thus, discovery of such a condition in one family member should raise the suspicion that it may exist in other family members. Congenitally absent teeth most commonly are third molars, second premolars, and lateral incisors.

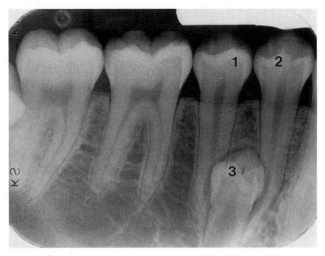

Figure 12–40. Supernumerary bicuspid in right mandible.

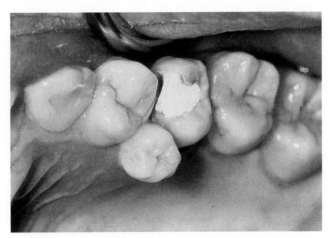

Figure 12–41. Maxillary supernumerary premolar that has erupted palatally in the arch.

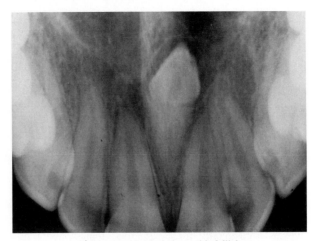

Figure 12–42. Mesiodens with follicle.

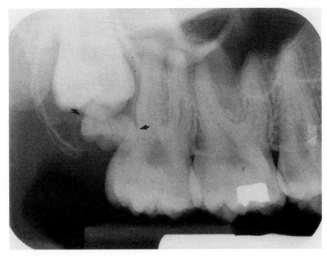

Figure 12–43. Supernumerary third molar *(arrows)* in the right maxilla.

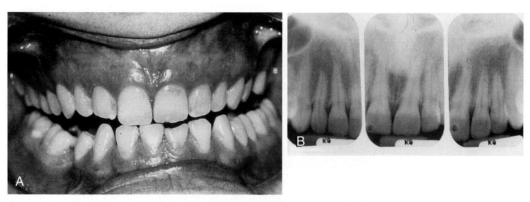

Figure 12–44. Example of bilateral supernumerary lateral incisors. *A*, Clinical photo of patient. *B*, Maxillary anterior periapical radiographs show the extra lateral incisors.

Figure 12–45 shows a relatively common finding in mixed dentitions. There is no evidence of a tooth or a developing follicle in the left quadrant beneath the mandibular second primary molar.

In contrast, the radiograph in Figure 12–46 shows a normally developing second bicuspid in a patient approximately 1 year older than the patient in Figure 12–45.

Also, in Figure 12–46 you should note the resorption of the distal root of the primary second molar. Succeeding permanent teeth "force" the primary teeth to exfoliate by causing root resorption. This is a normal physiologic process. Resorption may also occur pathologically, either as external or internal resorption. You will recall that Figure 12–6 in the section on trauma showed this process. That section differentiated normal apices from abnormal apices subjected to trauma. Figures 12–47, 12–48, and 12–49 show examples of root resorption and suggest their causes.

Discussion. Figures 12–47 and 12–48 show teeth that have undergone orthodontic movement. In most cases, the forces used in moving teeth cause no significant problems. However, occasionally forces are too great, moving teeth so quickly through the bone that external root resorption results.

Similarly, unerupted teeth, because of their eruptive potential (force) during root formation, can cause external resorption of adjacent roots—especially if the

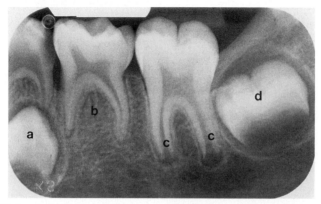

Figure 12–45. Developing first bicuspid *(a)*, lack of follicle for a second bicuspid *(b)*, developing apices of a permanent first molar *(c)*, and developing permanent second molar *(d)*.

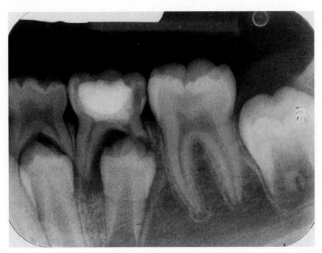

Figure 12–46. Normally developing dentition.

unerupted teeth are not in their normal positions for eruption. Figure 12–49 shows the consequence of not examining a patient radiographically to determine the reason for a tooth's absence in the mouth. This 55-year-old man will probably lose both bicuspids in this side of the mandible—teeth that would have made a more stable base for a lower partial denture.

Root resorption from trauma to the pulp may also be *iatrogenic*—that is, *caused by the operator.* Figure 12–50 shows an example of internal root resorption as a probable result. It also shows advanced, localized, periodontal bone destruction. The prognosis for this tooth is certain death.

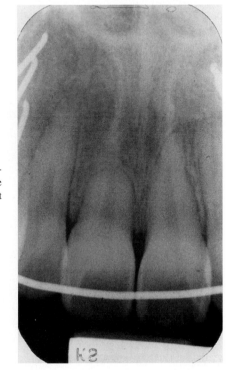

Figure 12–47. This patient is undergoing orthodontic tooth movement. The forces may have been excessive, which sometimes stimulates root resorption.

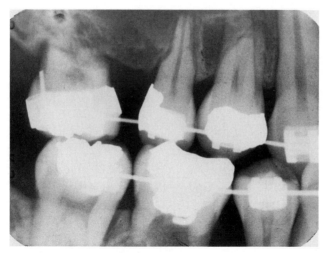

Figure 12–48. This patient also is undergoing orthodontic tooth movement. As seen in Figure 12–47, the forces may have been excessive, which sometimes stimulates root resorption.

Finally, teeth that have been impacted for many years sometimes become *ankylosed* (fused to the bone). The follicle around the crown of the tooth breaks down, and cells called *osteoclasts* may attack the bone and enamel to cause another type of external resorption. This process is seen in Figure 12–51. Figure 12–52, likewise, shows external resorption, bone replacement, and ankylosis. However, in this case the resorption was not preceded by breakdown of a follicle. The reason for the resorption is unknown, or *idiopathic*.

Another reactive process that causes changes to the root is the overproduction of cementum, termed *hypercementosis*. Most commonly, inflammation is the cause of this reaction; however, a tooth without an opposing "partner" with which to occlude may show hypercementosis. Figure 12–53 shows a radiographic and Figure 12–54 a clinical area of hypercementosis caused by inflammation, which also caused severe horizontal and vertical bone loss locally around the third molar.

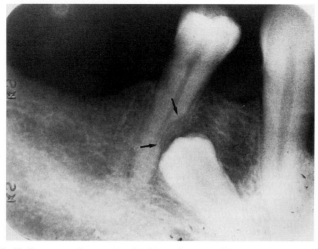

Figure 12–49. Root resorption as a result of force from an adjacent unerupted tooth *(arrows)*.

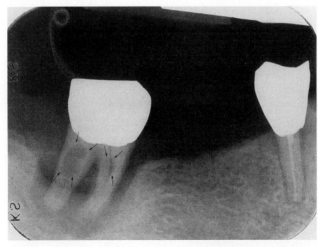

Figure 12–50. Internal resorption of both roots. These roots appear as enlargement of the pulp canal and are continuous with it.

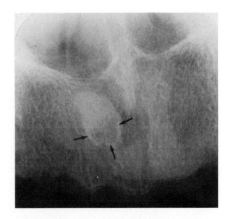

Figure 12–51. External resorption as a result of an impacted tooth *(arrows)* that has become anky-losed.

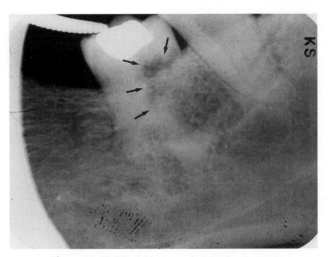

Figure 12–52. Idiopathic external resorption *(arrows)*.

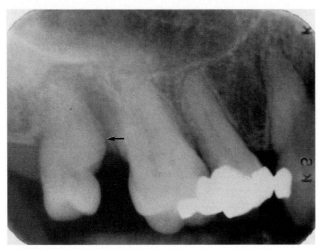

Figure 12–53. Hypercementosis resulting from inflammation. (Courtesy of Dr. John Lovas, Dalhousie University, Halifax, Nova Scotia.)

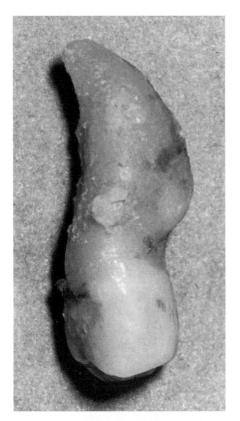

Figure 12–54. Hypercementosis resulting from inflammation. (Courtesy of Dr. John Lovas, Dalhousie University, Halifax, Nova Scotia.)

Figures 12–55 through 12–66 show some additional development abnormalities. They appear with brief descriptions.

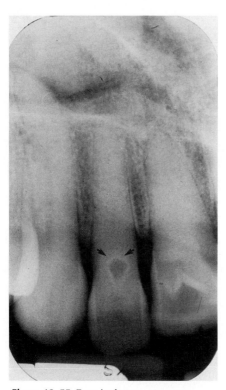

Dens in Dente. Tooth within a tooth. An inverted teardrop-shaped developmental pit lined with enamel, which can easily become decayed.

Figure 12–55. Dens in dente.

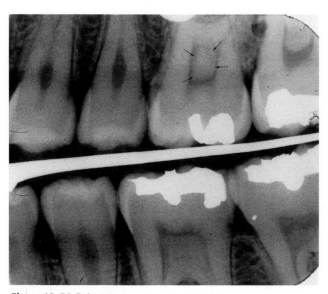

Pulp Stone. A *dystrophic* pulpal *calcification*, which can interfere with endodontic therapy. It occurs primarily in molar teeth; however, many other teeth in the dentition can show calcifications in pulp canals.

Figure 12–56. Pulp stone.

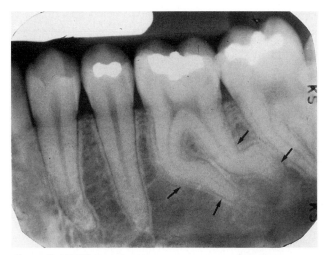

Figure 12–57. Dilacerated roots.

Dilacerated Root(s). *Severely curved roots.* These usually indicate that the tooth encountered some obstruction during the eruptive process. These roots are different from normally curved roots such as those of the maxillary lateral incisors and the lower third molars, with their distal curvatures. Teeth with dilacerated roots may be difficult to extract or to treat endodontically.

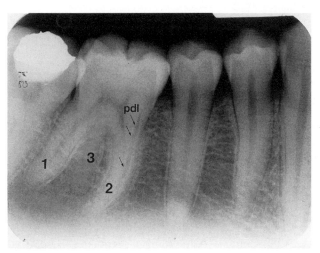

Figure 12–58. Multiple roots.

Multiple Roots. Canines, premolars, and molars can often have more roots than normal and, consequently, more pulpal canals. Note in Figure 12–58 that this molar has at least three roots. The arrows point to a periodontal ligament space *(pdl)* that appears "within" the mesial root; this root may also be divided.

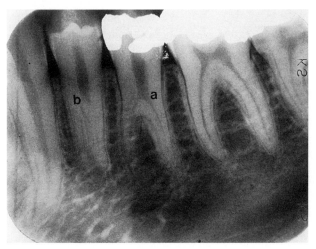

Figure 12–59. Taurodonts.

If a pulp chamber ends abruptly radiographically halfway down the root, then the canal has a *bifurcation*— either into *multiple roots* (Fig. 12–59, *a*) or simply within the same root (Fig. 12–59, *b*).

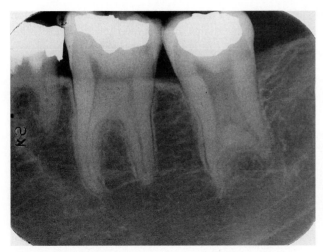

Figure 12–60. Taurodonts.

Taurodontism. Sometimes a tooth will have an elongated pulp chamber and short stubby roots, a condition called *taurodontism*. These teeth are termed *taurodonts* because their shape is "bull-like" (Fig. 12–60). Taurodontism can occur in primary teeth as well as in secondary teeth (Fig. 12–61). The tooth shown will probably require a pulpotomy.

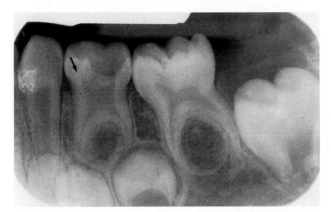

Figure 12–61. Taurodontism.

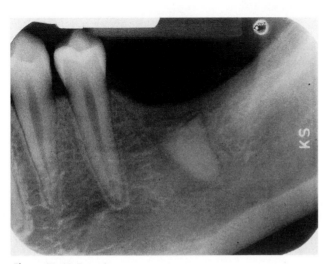

Figure 12–62. Root tips.

Root Tips. Root tips, or fragments of teeth, are sometimes left behind after difficult extractions. *They look like root tips* on a radiograph. Usually conical and found in former tooth locations, these fragments do not need to be removed unless they become secondarily infected. They should, however, be examined periodically using radiographs.

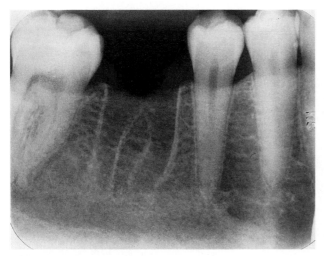

Figure 12–63. Extraction sites.

Extraction Sites. Recent extraction sites often show root "outlines"; this is due to the presence of the lamina dura around the tooth socket. The lamina dura usually disappears (remodels) within a few months. Socket sites, however, can take up to a year to heal and fill in.

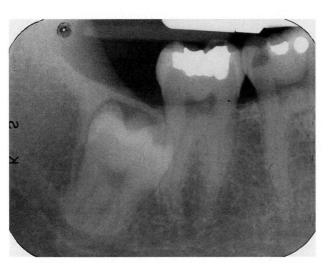

Figure 12–64. Mesioangular impaction of lower right permanent third molar.

Impacted Teeth. Figures 12–64 through 12–66 are examples of commonly impacted teeth, namely, third molars and maxillary cuspids.

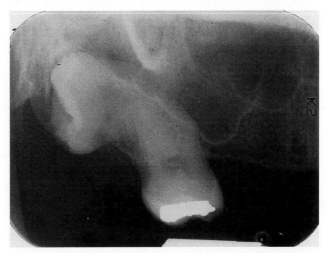

Figure 12–65. Horizontal impaction of maxillary right permanent third molar.

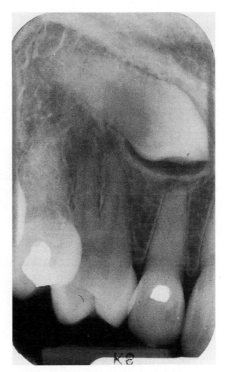

Figure 12–66. Maxillary right permanent cuspid impaction.

RADIOGRAPHIC FEATURES OF COMMON ORAL LESIONS

Figures 12–67 through 12–78 show some common radiographic appearances (presentations) of pathologic lesions. These appearances, or patterns, describe common radiologic features of lesions. This "pattern-matching" technique allows the clinician to categorize a lesion relatively quickly and then begin to formulate a differential diagnosis of the lesion based on its appearance, the clinical findings, and the patient's medical history. Radiographic examples of some of these patterns appear after the lists, along with line drawings for clarity and to allow comparison. A complete description of these lesions can be found in other radiology or pathology textbooks.

Common Radiographic Presentations of Various Odontogenic and Nonodontogenic Lesions

Periapical Radiolucencies

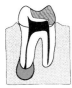

- Periapical abscess
- Periapical granuloma
- Periapical cyst
- Fibrous healing defect (surgical scar)
- Periapical cemental dysplasia (cementoma) (early stage)

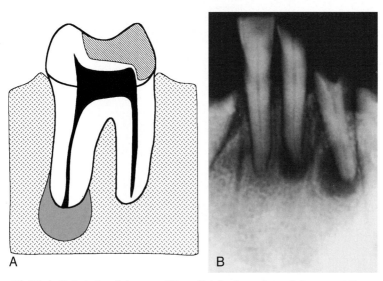

A   B

Figure 12–67. *A*, Periapical radiolucency. This well-defined, regular radiolucency at the apex of a lower molar represents an area termed *apical periodontitis*. This lesion histologically can be an abscess, a granuloma, or a cyst. It usually arises after the death of the pulp. Waste products from the necrotic pulp escape out of the apex and cause a biologic response that produces this appearance. *B*, Multiple well-defined radiolucencies secondary to severe dental caries. Each of these lesions could be termed apical periodontitis.

Radiolucencies with Distinct Borders

- Incisive canal cyst (nasopalatine duct cyst)
- Residual cyst
- Traumatic bone cyst
- Median palatal cyst
- Developmental lateral periodontal cyst

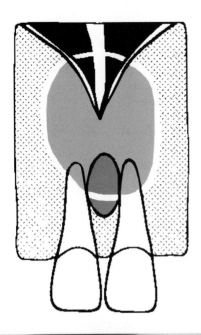

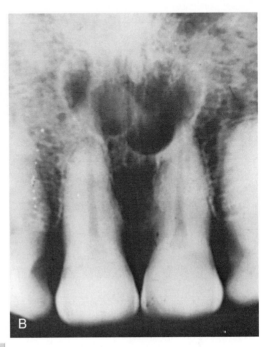

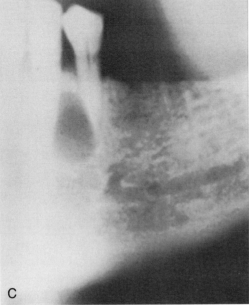

Figure 12–68. *A,* This large, expansile, well-defined radiolucency with a cortical (bony) outline between the central incisors suggests a cyst. The most common cyst of this region is called an *incisive canal cyst* or a *nasoalveolar duct cyst. B,* This well-defined, periapical, heart-shaped radiolucency is an incisive canal cyst. *C,* This radiograph shows a well-defined, unilocular radiolucency between two teeth. Both teeth were found to be vital. The lesion was a developmental, lateral periodontal cyst.

Radiolucencies with Indistinct Borders

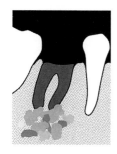

- Chronic osteomyelitis
- Osteosarcoma
- Chondrosarcoma
- Squamous cell carcinoma
- Metastatic tumors to the jaws
- Histiocytosis "X" (Langerhans' cell granuloma)
- Fibrous dysplasia
- Osteoradionecrosis

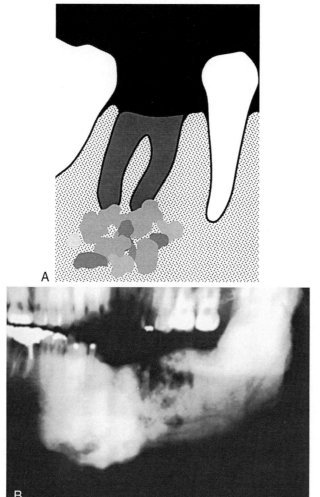

Figure 12–69. *A*, Radiolucency with indistinct borders. *B*, An ill-defined, mixed radiolucency-radiopacity consistent with an osteomyelitis infection.

Pericoronal Radiolucencies Without Calcifications

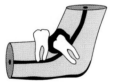

- Dentigerous cyst
- Ameloblastoma
- Odontogenic keratocyst
- Mucoepidermoid carcinoma
- Ameloblastic fibroma

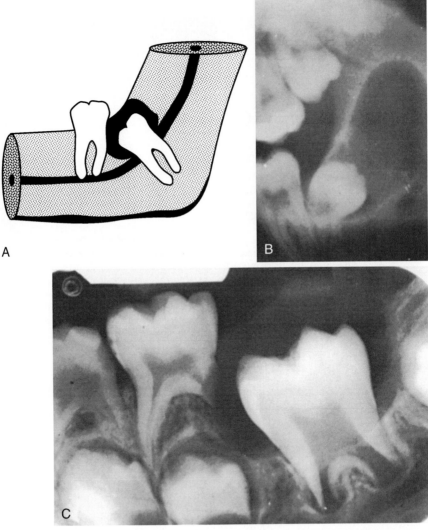

Figure 12–70. *A,* Pericoronal radiolucency without calcifications. This well-defined radiolucency surrounding the crown of a molar is termed a *pericoronal radiolucency.* Because the lesion contains no radiopacities, the differential diagnosis would include hyperplastic tooth follicle, ameloblastic fibroma, dentigerous cyst, or possibly odontogenic keratocyst or ameloblastoma. The last two lesions more commonly appear as *multilocular* lesions (see Fig. 12–71). *B,* A large, well-defined pericoronal radiolucency with a cortical border; it is probably a dentigerous cyst. *C,* A well-defined pericoronal radiolucency surrounding a developing first permanent molar, consistent with a hyperplastic tooth follicle.

Pericoronal Radiolucencies with Calcifications

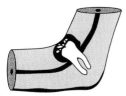

- Calcifying epithelial odontogenic tumor (Pindborg's tumor)
- Adenomatoid odontogenic tumor
- Calcifying odontogenic cyst (Gorlin's cyst)
- Ameloblastic fibro-odontoma
- Ameloblastic odontoma

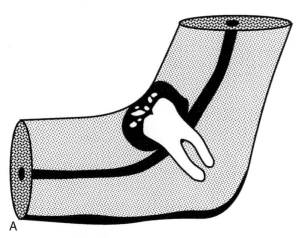 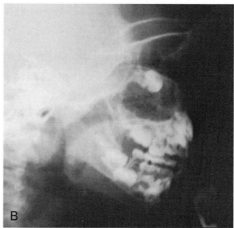

Figure 12–71. *A,* Pericoronal radiolucency with calcifications. This well-defined, pericoronal radiolucency differs from that shown in Figure 12–70*C* because it contains internal calcifications, or radiopacities. The differential diagnosis for lesions with this appearance can include calcifying epithelial odontogenic tumor (CEOT, Pindborg), calcifying odontogenic cyst (COC, Gorlin), adenomatoid odontogenic tumor (AOT), and ameloblastoma variants such as ameloblastic fibro-odontoma (AFO) or ameloblastic odontoma (AO). *B,* Ameloblastic fibro-odontoma in the maxillary sinus. (Courtesy of Dr. John Lovas, Dalhousie University, Halifax, Nova Scotia.)

Multilocular Radiolucencies

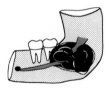

- Odontogenic keratocyst
- Ameloblastoma
- Central giant cell granuloma
- Aneurysmal bone cyst
- Hemangioma
- Fibrous dysplasia
- Cherubism (familial fibrous dysplasia)

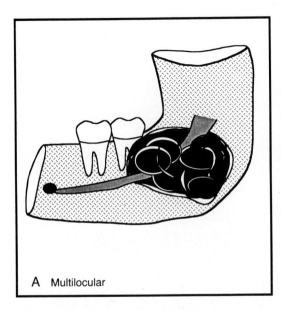

A Multilocular

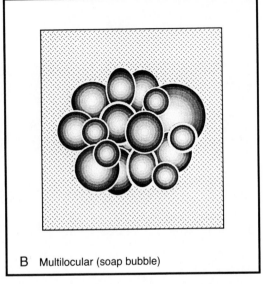

B Multilocular (soap bubble)

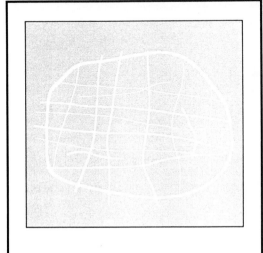

C Multilocular (tennis racket)

Figure 12–72. A, Multilocular radiolucency. This well-defined, multilocular radiolucent appearance can be ascribed to a number of lesions, including an ameloblastoma, an odontogenic keratocyst, a central giant cell granuloma, and others (see the list at the beginning of this section). Other multilocular appearances include "soap-bubble" and "tennis-racket" radiolucencies. Whereas soap-bubble radiolucencies are most commonly associated with ameloblastoma or odontogenic myxoma, the tennis-racket radiolucency is associated with vascular lesions such as aneurysmal bone cysts or hemangiomas. *B,* Schematic diagram of a multilocular (soap-bubble) radiolucency. *C,* Schematic diagram of a multilocular (tennis-racket) radiolucency.

Illustration continued on following page

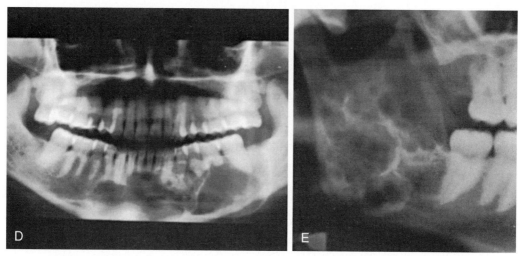

Figure 12–72 *Continued. D*, A large, expansile, multilocular lesion in the anterior mandible. It has a cortical outline and shows displaced teeth and resorbed root apices. Because it crosses the midline, it is suggestive of a central giant cell granuloma. *E*, A multilocular (soap-bubble) lesion in the right mandibular ramus. The patient had cherubism (familial fibrous dysplasia of jaw); the left ramus appeared identical.

Mixed Radiolucent-Radiopaque Lesions

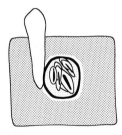

- Periapical cemental dysplasia (intermediate)
- Condensing osteitis
- Odontoma (compound and complex)
- Florid osseous dysplasia (gigantiform cementoma, diffuse sclerosing osteomyelitis)
- Cemento-ossifying fibroma
- Calcifying odontogenic cyst (Gorlin's cyst)
- Calcifying epithelial odontogenic tumor (Pindborg's tumor)
- Adenomatoid odontogenic tumor

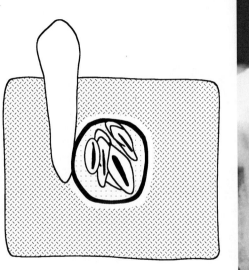

A

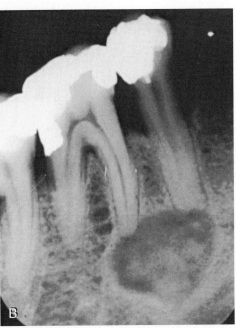

B

Figure 12–73. *A*, This well-defined, mixed radiolucent-radiopaque lesion represents a common tumor of odontogenic origin called an *odontoma*. The lesion is usually defined by a radiolucent rim, which is thought to represent a connective tissue "front." *B*, This mixed opacity at the apex of the molar is suggestive of a fibro-osseous lesion.

Periapical Radiopacities That May Contact Teeth

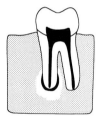

- Condensing osteitis
- Idiopathic osteosclerosis
- Periapical cemental dysplasia (mature)
- Hypercementosis
- Cementoblastoma
- Odontoma (complex or compound)

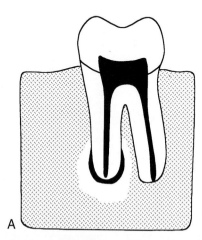

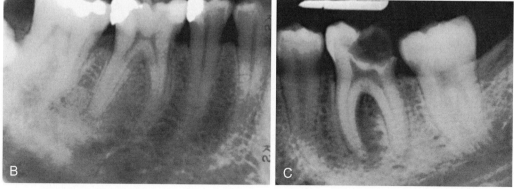

Figure 12–74. *A,* Periapical radiopacity. This well-defined radiopacity appears to blend into the surrounding bone. An area of radiolucency intervenes between the apex and the opacity. The lesion also has an irregular margin. The appearance is consistent with an area of condensing osteitis. Compare this diagram with the radiographic examples of the same lesion. Other periapical radiopacities include hypercementosis, osteosclerosis, and cementoblastoma. *B,* Condensing osteitis secondary to recurrent decay. Note how the lesion blends into the adjacent bone. Note also the altered trabecular pattern. *C,* Another example of condensing osteitis (sclerosing osteitis).

Solitary or Multiple Radiopacities Within the Jaws

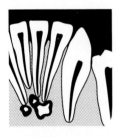

- Enostosis
- Exostosis
- Idiopathic osteosclerosis
- Periapical cemental dysplasia (mature)
- Retained root tip
- Odontoma

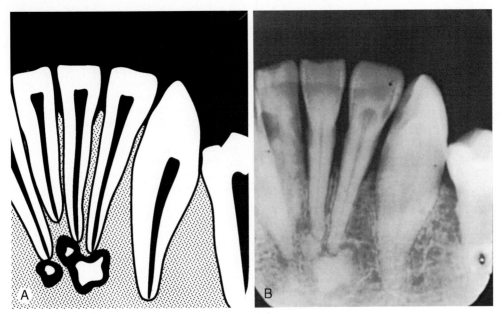

Figure 12–75. *A,* This diagram depicts multiple well-defined periapical radiopacities. The few lesions with this appearance include periapical cemental dysplasia (late or mature stage), florid osseous dysplasia (only one of several names), and possibly multiple osteomas (seen in Gardner's syndrome, although in Gardner's syndrome there would be no surrounding radiolucent rim). *B,* Periapical cemental dysplasia (late or mature stage).

Solitary or Multiple Radiopacities Outside the Jaws

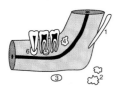

- Sialolith
- Antrolith
- Calcified lymph nodes
- Calcified stylohyoid ligament
- Calcified facial arteries

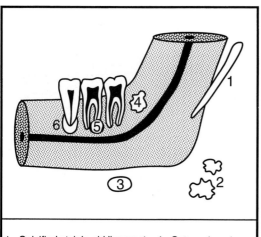

1. Calcified stylohyoid ligament
2. Calcified lymph nodes
3. Sialolith
4. Osteosclerosis
5. Cementoblastoma
6. Hypercementosis

Figure 12–76. Sometimes clinicians are confronted with radiopaque lesions outside the jaws. These lesions can include calcified lymph nodes, sialoliths, calcified blood vessels, and calcified stylohyoid ligaments, among others. This diagram depicts some of these lesions as well as some periapical radiopacities: *1*, calcified stylohyoid ligament; *2*, calcified lymph nodes; *3*, sialolith; *4*, osteosclerosis; *5*, cementoblastoma; and *6*, hypercementosis.

"Floating Tooth"

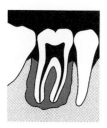

- Severe, localized periodontitis
- Juvenile periodontitis
- Eosinophilic granuloma (Langerhans' cell granuloma)
- Osteosarcoma
- Fibrosarcoma
- Lymphoma

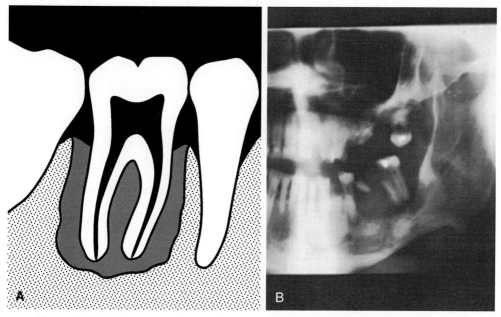

Figure 12–77. *A,* Diagram showing one of the more ominous radiographic appearances, the so-called *floating tooth.* The differential diagnosis for a floating tooth includes advanced periodontitis, juvenile periodontitis, eosinophilic granuloma (one of the histiocytosis X group, also called Langerhans' cell granuloma), and a sarcoma (osteo-, chondro-, or fibrosarcoma). *B,* Floating teeth in the mandibular left quadrant. A squamous cell carcinoma in the floor of the mouth involved the teeth and bone secondarily.

"Sun-Ray" Appearance

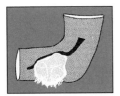

- Osteogenic sarcoma (classic)
- Hemangioma
- Chondrosarcoma
- Ameloblastic odontoma
- Complex odontoma

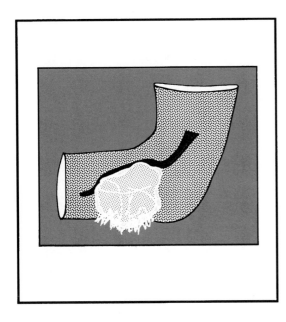

Figure 12–78. This diagram depicts the radiographic sign called a "sun-ray" effect. Bone trabeculae radiating at right angles from the affected bone are almost pathognomonic for an osteosarcoma.

Study Questions

1. Which of the following viewing strategies maximizes radiographic interpretation?
   A. Continuous eye movement.
   B. The use of a specific film sequence.
   C. Subdued lighting and a magnifying glass.
   D. Quiet surroundings without distractions.
   E. All of the above.
2. Which of these characteristics should you look for in determining normal versus abnormal radiographs?
   A. Asymmetry of structures.
   B. Breaks in continuity.
   C. Change in dimension.
   D. All of the above.
3. An interproximal caries often appears as a
   A. Radiopaque extension, or "spur."
   B. Radiolucent line around the root of the tooth.
   C. Moon- or wedge-shaped radiolucency.
   D. Moon- or wedge-shaped radiopacity.
4. An interproximal caries is frequently found in which area of the tooth?
   A. Just apical to the pulp chamber.
   B. At or slightly coronal to the contact point.
   C. At or slightly apical to the contact point.
   D. Just apical to the central occlusal pit.
5. A root surface caries on the mesial or distal aspect of a periodontally involved tooth is frequently found
   A. Apical to the CEJ.
   B. Coronal to the CEJ.
   C. At the apex of the root.
   D. Apical to the alveolar crest.
6. What characteristics of a root caries differ from those of other interproximal caries?
   A. The location on the tooth.
   B. The shape of the lesion.
   C. The radiographic classification.
   D. All of the above.
7. Which of the following is not classified as a developmental dental abnormality?
   A. Taurodont.
   B. Mesiodens.
   C. Dens in dente.
   D. Periapical abscess.
8. Which of the following has a radiopaque appearance?
   A. Periapical cyst.
   B. Mandibular torus.
   C. Dentigerous cyst.
   D. Ameloblastoma.

9. The term *pericoronal* means
    A. At the apex of a root.
    B. Around the root of a tooth.
    C. Around the crown of a tooth.
    D. Around the periodontal ligament space.
10. The term *multilocular* refers to a radiographic appearance that may resemble which of the following?
    A. A piece of cotton.
    B. The rays of the sun.
    C. A group of soap bubbles.
    D. An orange peel.

Chapter 13

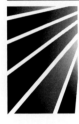

Radiation Biology and Protection

You will frequently hear from your patients, "I've heard x rays are bad for me. Do you really need to take them?" Aside from educating your patients about the diagnostic importance of dental radiographs, you will have to address their fears of radiation. What will you tell them? What do you, as a person working with radiation, need to know about it?

The science of the effects of radiation on living organisms is called *radiation biology*. This chapter discusses these effects as they apply to the biologic molecules and cells of the body. It also discusses how much radiation is received from dental radiographs, the risks that are involved with these exposures, and how to protect yourself and your patient from unnecessary or excess radiation.

MOLECULAR CHANGES

As a beam of radiation passes through matter, it gradually weakens and eventually disappears. The energy of the beam is transferred to the material through which it passes. This transfer of energy is called *absorption*.

Direct Effects

Interaction of X Rays and Molecules

Diagnostic x radiation interacts with matter at the atomic level in body tissues in three ways. These interactions are called *classical scattering,* the *photoelectric effect,* and the *Compton effect* (Fig. 13–1).

Classical Scattering (Coherent Scattering, Thompson Effect). When a low-energy x-ray photon approaches an outer orbital electron of an atom, it may not have enough energy to eject the electron from its orbit. Instead, the photon may interact with the electron and cause it to be "excited," or to vibrate. The photon "transfers" all of its energy to the excited electron, and the photon ceases to exist. The vibrating electron then radiates its acquired energy in the form of another x-ray photon with the same energy level as the first photon. The new photon exits the atom, usually in a different direction. The radiation, then, has "scattered." In diagnostic radiology, little of this classical scattering occurs (Fig. 13–1A).

Photoelectric Effect. The photoelectric interaction occurs when an x-ray photon of sufficient energy collides with an inner orbiting electron in an atom. All of the energy from the photon is used to eject the electron from its orbit, and the photon ceases to exist. The atom absorbs the radiation with no scatter. The ejected electron speeds away as a *recoil electron.*

When the atom loses one of its inner electrons, one of the electrons in an outer orbit drops down to fill the vacancy left by the recoil electron. When the outer electron moves to another level in the atom, energy is given off in the form of an

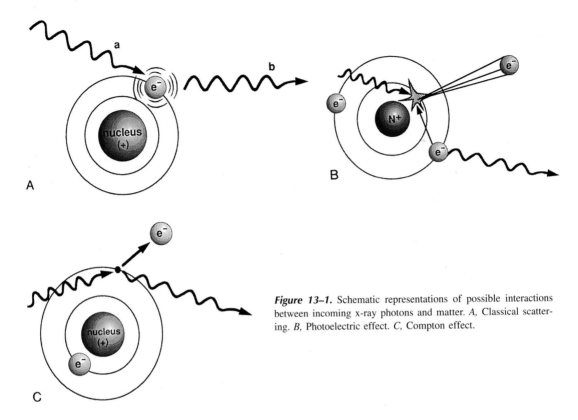

Figure 13–1. Schematic representations of possible interactions between incoming x-ray photons and matter. *A,* Classical scattering. *B,* Photoelectric effect. *C,* Compton effect.

x-ray photon. Each orbit of every type of atom has a specific energy level, and the photon that is generated in this process will have that specific energy.

The atom is still missing one electron and thus has a net positive charge. Such an atom, called an *ion,* can interact with other atoms and molecules (Fig. 13–1*B*).

Compton Effect. The Compton effect occurs when a photon with sufficient energy collides with an outer orbital electron in an atom, ejecting it from its orbit. In this instance, however, the incoming photon does not transfer all of its energy to the recoil electron, but continues in a different direction as a photon with lower energy. The energy of the photon equals the energy of the incident (incoming) photon minus the energy used to eject the electron. Therefore, the Compton effect results in energy absorption by the atom, ionization of the atom, and the release of scatter radiation. The Compton effect and the photoelectric effect occur in nearly equal proportions in dental radiography (Fig. 13–1*C*).

The ionized atoms and the recoil electrons of the photoelectric effect and the Compton effect may cause further molecular interactions in the patient's tissues. These *direct effects* of radiation may result in

1. Breaking molecules into smaller pieces.
2. Disrupting molecular bonds.
3. Forming new bonds within molecules.
4. Forming new bonds between molecules.

Indirect Effects

Molecules not directly affected by x rays can be altered indirectly. Living organisms consist mostly of water. If an x-ray photon interacts with water and oxygen, compounds called *free radicals* are formed. The process is called *radiolysis*. A free radical readily reacts with other biologic molecules. Radicals may remove electrons or hydrogen atoms from organic molecules, add bonds, or initiate intermolecular bonding. Examples of radicals created by the radiolysis of water include

$$x\text{-ray photon} \rightarrow H_2O \rightarrow H^{\cdot} + OH^{\cdot} \text{ (hydrogen radical + hydroxyl radical)}$$
$$H^{\cdot} + O_2 \rightarrow HO_2^{\cdot} \text{ (peroxyl radical)}$$

In addition, two hydroxyl radicals ($OH^{\cdot}$) can combine to form hydrogen peroxide (H_2O_2), a chemical toxic to most cells. The reaction would appear as

$$OH^{\cdot} + OH^{\cdot} \rightarrow H_2O_2 \text{ (hydrogen peroxide)}$$

An organic molecule (RH) could be altered as follows:

$$RH + H^{\cdot} \rightarrow R^{\cdot} + H_2$$
$$RH + OH^{\cdot} \rightarrow R^{\cdot} + H_2O$$

The effects caused by the radicals are not directly the result of a molecule being "hit" by radiation. Because the damage is mediated by a free radical, it is referred to as an *indirect effect* of radiation. The indirect actions of x rays can damage biologic molecules as easily as can the direct actions. In fact, indirect effects have a higher probability of causing biologic damage than do direct effects. Any changes in an organic molecule, no matter how the molecule is damaged, may result in altered cell function. In summary, indirect effects of radiation include (1) the production of free radicals, which in turn causes (2) the alteration of other molecules. Free radical production in the body can have causes other than x radiation: chemicals in food, exposure to the sun, and toxins in the air that are breathed into the body.

CELLULAR EFFECTS

A cell has two basic components, the nucleus and the cytoplasm. Ionizing radiation may affect either area or both. Damage in the nucleus often affects the chromosomes, which contain DNA (deoxyribonucleic acid). The DNA in each organism is composed of a particular series of bases. The specific order of the DNA bases is the foundation for the genetic code, making each organism unique. Radiation may alter the base sequence of the DNA molecule and make it defective (Fig. 13–2).

Defective DNA may lead to the disruption of the mechanisms for cell division (mitosis). There may be delayed cell division or loss of reproductive capacity of the cells. Errors that are permanently incorporated into the DNA are passed on to future generations of the affected cells as *mutations*. If the defective DNA is contained in a reproductive cell (sperm or ovum), then the defect may be passed along to future generations of organisms. This, then, would be a *genetic effect* of radiation.

Radiation can also affect cellular cytoplasm. Cells may develop the following problems if the cytoplasm is damaged:

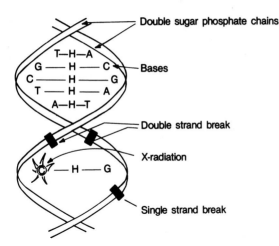

Figure 13–2. X-ray interaction occurs as a "hit" on the "target" DNA molecule. The hit damages a portion of the molecule (and thus the genetic code). The damaged base sequence may be improperly repaired or replaced by a different sequence. (Adapted from Kasle MJ and Langlais RP: Basic Principles of Oral Radiography, vol. 4. Philadelphia: WB Saunders Company, 1981, p. 138.)

1. Increased permeability or rupture of membranes.
2. Nonfunctional organelles such as lysosomes, endoplasmic reticulum, and mitochondria.
3. Inactivation of enzymes.
4. Coagulation of the cytoplasmic fluid.

Any one of these changes could result in the disruption of cell function or even in cell death.

All body tissues except the reproductive cells are called *somatic tissues.* The *somatic effects* of radiation may occur in the cell cytoplasm or nucleus. If the damage to the cells is severe enough, the organism may become ill or even die. However, somatic effects of radiation are *not* passed along to future generations, the way genetic effects are. Genetic effects occur only in the reproductive cells.

Cellular Sensitivity to Radiation

Some cells are more sensitive to radiation than others. A cell will be more sensitive to radiation if it has any of the following characteristics:

1. High mitotic rate (it undergoes frequent cell divisions).
2. Long mitotic history (it undergoes many divisions over time).
3. Primitive or immature nature (it must undergo further growth or development).
4. Undifferentiated nature (it is not highly specialized).

An exception is the *lymphocyte,* which is a highly specialized cell that is part of the immune system. It will not divide once it is mature. The **small lymphocyte** is probably the **cell most sensitive to radiation.** Table 13–1 lists various groups of cells and their relative radiation sensitivity.

SHORT- AND LONG-TERM EFFECTS OF RADIATION

Harmful effects of radiation do not show up immediately. A time lag exists between exposure to radiation and the signs and symptoms of biologic damage.

TABLE 13–1. RELATIVE RADIATION SENSITIVITY OF CELLS AND TISSUES

SENSITIVITY TO RADIATION	CELL TYPE OR TISSUE
High	Small lymphocyte
	Bone marrow
	Reproductive cells
	Intestinal mucosa
Fairly high	Skin
	Lens of the eye
	Oral mucosa
Medium	Connective tissue
	Small blood vessels
	Growing bone and cartilage
Fairly low	Mature bone and cartilage
	Salivary gland
	Thyroid gland
	Kidney
	Liver
Low	Muscle
	Nerve

This period of time, called the *latent period,* may be as short as a few hours or as long as 20 years or more. The length of the latent period depends on the total dose of radiation received and the amount of time it took to receive that dose. The higher the dose and the shorter the dose rate, the shorter the latent period is.

Short-term, or acute, effects of radiation usually result from high doses to the entire body. Symptoms may include nausea, vomiting, diarrhea, fever, loss of hair, hemorrhage, and even total body collapse. Long-term, or chronic, effects of radiation are usually the result of doses of radiation received over a long period of time. The effects may not be seen for several months or even years.

Repeated radiation exposure produces *cumulative effects.* Tissues have the capacity to repair radiation damage to a certain degree; however, some damage cannot be repaired and accumulates in the tissues. In other words, **radiation itself does not accumulate, but some of the unrepaired damage might.** Thus, one acute exposure of 10 R (R = roentgen; see the explanation of units provided later) would be more biologically damaging than 10 exposures of 1 R spread over 10 years, even though the total dosage for each is 10 R. Unrepaired damage can lead to future health problems such as the development of cancer, cataracts, birth defects, or premature aging. Table 13–2 lists tissues and organs considered "critical organs" that might be affected by dental x radiation. This chapter discusses some of these critical organs later.

At one time it was believed that very low doses of radiation were not harmful to patients. It was thought that there was a certain threshold below which no

TABLE 13–2. CUMULATIVE EFFECT OF REPEATED EXPOSURE (ORGAN AND DISORDER)

CRITICAL ORGAN	RESULTING DISORDER
Lens of eye	Cataracts
Bone marrow	Leukemia
Salivary gland	Cancer
Thyroid gland	Cancer
Skin	Cancer
Gonads	Genetic abnormalities

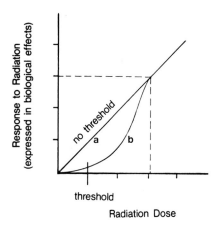

Figure 13–3. The diagonal, straight line *a* represents the extrapolation of damage owing to low doses of x radiation in a nonthreshold manner; that is, any amount of radiation will cause some damage. Curve *b* represents a nonlinear threshold approach in which a certain radiation dose must be received before damage can be observed.

biologic damage occurred (Fig. 13–3). It now appears that there is no safe level of radiation. The low doses received by the patient from dental radiography produce very little damage, but damage does occur. The number of cells in the body that are affected is low, and the probability of cell death is even lower. Nevertheless, it is necessary to keep exposure to x radiation to a minimum.

UNITS OF RADIATION MEASUREMENT

Before we can discuss the amounts of radiation associated with dental films, we must define the way radiation is measured. To complicate matters, two sets of terminology are currently in use. In 1985 an international system (SI) of measurement was adopted worldwide. However, "traditional" terminology was used in older textbooks and journals. Both systems are presented here.

The amount of radiation a person is exposed to is measured in SI units as coulombs per kilogram. This is a measure of electric charge in a certain mass of air. Most people find it more convenient to use the "old" term, the *roentgen* (abbreviated as R). The roentgen is the unit of radiation exposure that produces one electrostatic charge per cubic centimeter of air.

The amount of radiation energy actually absorbed by the tissues is the *absorbed dose*. The SI unit of absorbed dose is called a *gray* (Gy). It is defined as the transfer of 10 joules (a unit of energy and work) per kilogram of tissue. The traditional system uses the term *rad* (*r*adiation *a*bsorbed *d*ose) as the unit of measurement. One rad is equivalent to the transfer of 100 *ergs* (another unit of energy and work) per gram of tissue; 1 gray (Gy) equals 100 rad.

Traditionally, the *rem* (*r*oentgen-*e*quivalent-*m*an) is the unit of dose equivalence.

TABLE 13–3. UNITS OF RADIATION MEASUREMENT

QUANTITY	SI UNITS	TRADITIONAL UNITS	CONVERSION
Exposure	Coulombs per kilograms (C/kg)	Roentgen (R)	1 C/kg = 3880 R
Dose	Gray (Gy)	Rad	1 Gy = 100 rad
Dose equivalence	Sievert (Sv)	Rem	1 Sv = 100 rems

It is defined as the absorbed dose of any form of radiation that produces the same biologic effect in a human as does 1.0 rad of x radiation. Different forms of ionizing radiation have different energies. One rem of x radiation has a different amount of energy than 1 rem of α-particle radiation. Yet they will both produce the same effects in a human. The SI unit of dose equivalence is the *sievert* (Sv); 1 sievert (Sv) equals 100 rems.

Technically, some differences exist between the units of radiation measurement, but in dental radiology the units are virtually interchangeable.

$$1 \text{ roentgen (R)} = 1 \text{ rad} = 1 \text{ rem}$$

and

$$1 \text{ gray (Gy)} = 1 \text{ sievert (Sv) in SI units}$$

The amounts of radiation involved in dental radiography are much smaller than 1 Gy or 1 Sv. Just as a meter can be divided into centimeters or millimeters, the units of radiation measurement can be divided. For example, a *centi*gray is one-hundredth of a gray (abbreviated cGy), a *milli*rad is one-thousandth of a rad (abbreviated mrad), and a *micro*sievert is one-millionth of a sievert (abbreviated μSv). Table 13–3 gives a summary of the units of radiation measurement.

AMOUNTS OF RADIATION USED IN DENTAL RADIOGRAPHY

The exact amount of radiation exposure produced when taking dental radiographs varies, depending on film speed, technique used, kilovoltage used, and whether any additional collimation is present. Speed "E" film requires only about one-third to one-half as much radiation for a diagnostic image as does speed "D" film. Higher kilovoltages and longer source-to-film distances (SFD) result in lower skin doses than do lower kilovoltages and shorter distances. Rectangular collimation further reduces the amount of tissue exposed to the x-ray beam by about 60 percent to 70 percent. Table 13–4 lists various exposures to skin with different kilovoltages and SFDs.

Techniques that employ intensifying screens generally require less radiation. The exposures in panoramic radiography vary from site to site, but they are often not higher than 200 μGy to 300 μGy. In fact, for many areas of the head and

TABLE 13–4. RADIATION EXPOSURES TO SKIN DURING INTRAORAL RADIOGRAPHY

	70 kVp* 16-INCH SFD**	90 kVp* 16-INCH SFD**	70 kVp* 8-INCH SFD**	90 kVp* 8-INCH SFD**
Single Film	250 mR (2.5 mGy)†	175 mR (1.75 mGy)†	375 mR (3.75 mGy)†	275 mR (2.75 mGy)†
18-Film Series	4500 mR (45 mGy)†	3150 mR (31.5 mGy)†	6750 mR (67.5 mGy)†	4950 mR (49.5 mGy)†

* kVp = kilovolt peak; values are for speed "D" film.
† The milligray (mGy) is not a unit for exposure, but the authors find coulombs per kilogram (C/kg) a cumbersome unit. The SI unit is included for comparison and completeness.
** SFD = source-to-film distance.

TABLE 13–5. ABSORBED DOSES TO MANDIBULAR BONE MARROW

PANORAMIC FILMS	CMRS*		PBW†	
	RECTANGULAR COLLIMATION	*ROUND COLLIMATION*	*RECTANGULAR COLLIMATION*	*ROUND COLLIMATION*
600 μGy	2500 μGy	7000 μGy	500 μGy	2500 μGy

* 20-film complete mouth radiographic survey.
† 4 films.

neck, the dose is less than 50 μGy. The absorbed skin doses associated with skull films are only about 5 μGy. Absorbed doses to the bone marrow and other deeper structures are lower than the skin doses with all techniques. Table 13–5 gives examples of doses to bone marrow associated with dental radiography.

RISK VERSUS BENEFIT OF DENTAL FILMS

We are exposed to radiation every day of our lives. Background radiation comes from natural sources such as radioactive materials in the ground and cosmic radiation from space. It also comes from man-made sources such as radioactive waste and nuclear fallout. The average background radiation for the U.S. population is approximately 1.0 to 1.8 millisieverts (mSv) per year; it varies slightly with geographic location. Some areas contain more radioactive materials in the ground: areas of higher elevation, such as Denver, Colorado, receive more cosmic radiation. The background exposure does not include the radiation from medical or dental sources or from consumer goods and activities.

Critical Organs

Although the radiation doses from dental radiography are small, there is a potential for biologic damage every time tissues are exposed to radiation. Some tissues or organs are exposed to more radiation than others when dental films are taken. If these tissues are damaged, the quality of an individual's life declines. These tissues or organs are the *critical organs.*

The **skin** is the first tissue exposed to radiation from sources outside the body. One of its responses to radiation exposure is a reddening, or an erythema. This is the same reaction seen in a sunburn. (Remember that sunlight is also a form of electromagnetic radiation.) Exposure to radiation increases the risk of skin cancer. Yet increased risks for skin cancer have not been shown with doses of x radiation less than 250 mGy. The dose to the skin of the face is about 10 mGy when the operator takes dental films using an open-ended cylinder and speed "D" film, and the dose is substantially reduced with speed "E" film and rectangular collimation. Therefore, a patient would have to receive at least 25 complete mouth radiographic series (CMRS) in a very short time to significantly increase the risk of skin cancer.

Radiation to the **lens of the eye** may produce cataracts (a cloudiness of the lens). The x-ray dose associated with this problem appears to be about 2 Gy (2,000 mGy). The dose to the eye from a CMRS, using an open-ended cylinder and speed

"D" film, is only about 0.6 mGy. Many scientists no longer consider the eye lens a critical organ.

The **thyroid gland** is fairly resistant to radiation in the adult. However, thyroid cancer has been found in people who were exposed to a dose as low as 50 mGy (500,000 µGy) when they were children. The dose to the thyroid from a CMRS (open-ended rectangle, speed "E" film) is less than 300 µGy. This dose to the thyroid can be further reduced by about half with the use of a thyroid collar.

Malignant changes in **bone marrow** may result in leukemia. There is active (blood-cell-producing) marrow in the mandible, skull, and cervical spine. About 13 percent of the total bone marrow lies in the head and neck areas. The dose to the bone marrow in a full mouth series of radiographs (open-ended rectangle, speed "E" film) is about 2,500 µGy. The x-ray dose associated with leukemia is about 50 mGy.

As we have learned, the genetic effects of radiation can have far-reaching results. However, the dose to the **reproductive cells** from dental radiography is *very* small: only about 50 µGy or less for males and 30 µGy for females. The female dose is lower because the reproductive cells are in a more protected body location. If the patient wears a lead apron, exposure to the reproductive cells is virtually zero (1.0 µGy to 3.0 µGy).

The exact amount of x radiation that may produce damage to a developing human **embryo** or **fetus** is unknown. It is thought that doses below 10,000 µGy produce very little risk. However, to preserve the woman's peace of mind, some practitioners prefer to postpone nonemergency radiographs until after the delivery. For urgent care, a minimal number of films can be taken using standard radiation protection practices.

In summary, there is some risk attached to the use of ionizing radiation on biologic tissues. Table 13–6 lists estimates of the probabilities of finding excess fatal cancers associated with dental radiography in a large population. Still, the levels of radiation involved in dental radiography are only about one twenty-fifth to one one-thousandth of the levels associated with injury. Therefore, the benefit of detecting disease in a patient—disease that might not otherwise be detected—far outweighs the risks of receiving small doses of radiation, if the radiographs are prescribed and are exposed and processed in an appropriate manner.

TABLE 13–6. PROBABILITY OF EXCESS FATAL CANCERS PER MILLION RADIOGRAPHIC EXAMS

RADIOGRAPHIC SURVEY	FILM SPEED AND COLLIMATION	NUMBER OF EXCESS CANCERS
Posterior bitewings (4 films)	"D" speed film Round collimation	30
	"E" speed film Round collimation	27
	"E" speed film Rectangular collimation	4
Complete mouth survey (CMRS) (20 films)	"D" speed film Round collimation	75
	"E" speed film Round collimation	48
	"E" speed film Rectangular collimation	26

RADIATION PROTECTION FOR THE PATIENT

Despite the low risks to the patient from dental radiography, it is best to keep exposure to ionizing radiation to a minimum. Therefore, the *ALARA* concept should be kept in mind when exposing dental films: "*As Low As Reasonably Achievable*." Remember, *you* control the amount of radiation your patient receives, and that exposure should be kept as low as possible. Following are some ways to adhere to the ALARA concept:

Film Selection. Fast film should be used; at least speed "D" for bitewings and periapicals. Speed "E" film further reduces patient exposure by at least 40 percent and perhaps as much as 50 percent. *Selection criteria* for the number and types of films should be used by the clinician to minimize exposure. The prescribing of radiographs for specific reasons rather than using them routinely is an effective method of reducing x-radiation doses. This concept is known as using selection criteria.

Kilovoltage. Using an x-ray beam with low kilovoltage results in higher patient doses, primarily to the skin. The lower-energy x-ray photons are absorbed by the patient's tissues. They do not reach the film and therefore do not contribute to the diagnostic image. Units should be operated using *at least* 60 kVp and preferably an even higher setting.

Filtration. Units operating at 70 kVp or above should have filtration equivalent to 2.5 mm of aluminum. Units operating below 70 kVp should have the equivalent of 1.5 mm of aluminum. Filtration removes the low-energy x rays from the beam. These "soft" x rays are absorbed by the patient and do not contribute to the image; removing them before they reach the patient reduces radiation exposure.

X-Ray Beam Collimation. The beam should be collimated so that it is no more than 7 cm (2.75 inches) in diameter at the patient's face. Rectangular collimation further reduces the amount of tissue irradiated because of the reduced area of skin surface exposed and the reduction in the number of overlapping fields. Rectangular collimation can result in a dose reduction of 50 percent to 90 percent, depending on the anatomic site being radiographed.

Position-Indicating Devices. Open-ended, circular, or rectangular lead-lined cylinders are preferred for directing the x-ray beam. A long (12- to 16-inch) position-indicating device (PID) will reduce exposure to the patient better than a short (8-inch) PID, because there will be less divergence of the beam. *Pointed plastic cones are NOT recommended and are illegal in some states:* the x rays interact with the plastic and increase the amount of *scatter radiation* produced (Fig. 13–4).

Technique. The use of film-holding devices is recommended. These devices usually result in a more stable positioning of the film. In addition, the patient's hands are not exposed to radiation. If rectangular collimation is being used, a film holder with a positioning guide is necessary.

Retakes should be kept to a minimum. If you are in doubt about the placement of a film or the position of the tubehead, *do not press the exposure button*. Be sure you are taking the best film that you can.

Patients should be observed at all times during film exposure.

Proper Processing. The best technique in the world will not produce films of good quality if your processing standards are not acceptable. A quality assurance program such as the one outlined in Chapter 2 will help to ensure that film processing is adequate.

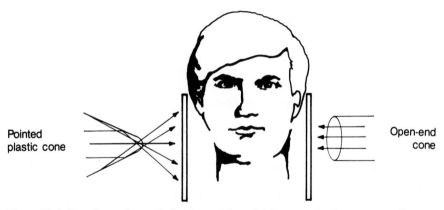

Figure 13–4. X-ray interactions with the slopes of the pointed cone scatter the more energetic x rays in a wider pattern, resulting in a greater skin-surface radiation dose.

Miscellaneous. *Lead aprons should be used on all patients.* Thyroid collars should be used on patients when intraoral films are being taken. Sound professional judgment can help minimize patient exposures; the minimum number of films that cover the areas desired should be used. "Routine" films taken at predetermined time intervals are *not* recommended. Clinicians should always specify a reason for the films they order based on the subjective complaints of and objective signs in their patients. **Selection Criteria** can be used to prescribe the type and number of radiographs required.

RADIATION PROTECTION FOR THE OPERATOR

People who work with radiation are entitled to protection from radiation. Exposure limits have been established for occupationally exposed workers. The *maximum permissible dose* (MPD) is the dose of radiation to the whole body that produces very little chance of somatic or genetic injury. The current MPD for whole-body exposure per year for occupationally exposed personnel is 0.05 Sv (5.0 rem). However, consideration is being given to lowering the dose to 0.02 Sv. An age-based formula has also been developed as a guideline for any accumulated dose (N = age in years):

$$MPD = 50mSv \times N$$

Occupationally exposed women who are pregnant are allowed an MPD of only 0.005 Sv per year. This is the same dose limit that applies to the general population. Therefore, during their pregnancies, female radiation workers should be treated like the general population and should receive far less radiation than the occupationally exposed group.

A film badge service is a good way to keep track of occupational exposure. Badges are worn by personnel at all times while at work. The badges are regularly sent to the company providing the exposure measurement service. Written reports of the exposure recorded on the badges are provided. If proper safety precautions are followed, no one in a dental office should receive radiation doses close to their MPD.

It is preferable that the operator stand behind an appropriate barrier while exposing films. The barrier should have a window or other means of monitoring the patient during the exposure. If no barrier is available, the operator should stand at least 6 feet away from the patient and in an area that lies between 90 degrees and 135 degrees to the primary x-ray beam. These are areas of minimum scatter radiation (see Chapter 1 to review these areas).

Dental personnel should *never* hold films for patients. If assistance is necessary, ask a family member or guardian to help. Be sure to protect the helper with a lead apron. Dental personnel should *never* hold the tubehead for stability. If the equipment is that unstable, *it should not be used until it is professionally repaired.*

The operatory that contains the x-ray unit should be constructed so that it protects the people in surrounding areas from radiation. Most dental offices have a fairly low radiation workload. This means that low milliamperage and exposure times are used. Shielding or barrier requirements are based on workload, kilovoltages used, distances involved, and an occupancy factor (who is in the area and how often). Regular construction materials such as plaster, cinderblock, and at least 2½ inches of drywall will provide adequate protection from the radiation produced by dental units. Wood paneling alone does not provide adequate protection. It should be backed with additional materials to provide a safe environment for everyone. Guidelines for barrier construction may be found in the NCRPM (National Council on Radiation Protection and Measurements) publication no. 35.

LEGAL ASPECTS OF DENTAL RADIOGRAPHY

Liability has become a major concern in all service industries. Proceeding with ignorance, carelessness, lack of professional skill, or disregard for established rules or principles constitutes malpractice. The following discussion addresses these issues.

The decision to obtain dental radiographs for a patient and the number and types of radiographs to be obtained are to be determined by a licensed dentist, or a properly supervised dental student, as part of his or her contractual duty to the patient. The decision to order radiographs must be based on the idea that the benefit derived from the diagnostic radiograph outweighs the risk to the patient. This concept is termed "selection criteria" and has been adopted by most major specialty groups in the United States and Canada as well as by the American and Canadian Dental Associations.

The decision whether to order radiographs cannot be reasonably accomplished without first obtaining a radiation history of the patient to determine if there are contraindications. The information obtained should contribute significantly to the proper diagnosis, treatment, and prevention of disease. This guideline indicates that each patient should be evaluated clinically to determine the need for radiographs. Taking radiographs based on a predetermined timetable is not accepted as the standard of care. Just as taking radiographs that are not necessary is unsound practice, so is providing treatment without radiographs that are needed for quality care. Both situations may be considered malpractice. In addition, films that are not diagnostically usable are also a source of malpractice.

The 1981 Consumer-Patient Radiation Health and Safety Act addresses the legal responsibility for quality and maintenance of equipment, certification of all persons using ionizing radiation equipment, and the accreditation of education programs to train such personnel. The act states that equipment must be properly maintained and must be inspected regularly, according to state statutes. It also leaves the dentist to assume vicarious liability for the radiographic services provided by his or her employees. Using operators that are not certified leaves both the employee and the employer open to legal problems of statute violations and malpractice. All employees exposing patients to ionizing radiation must be verified as competent in technique and protection procedures.

Before exposing any patient to ionizing radiation, the operator must receive documented "informed consent" from the patient. In order to receive this consent, it is necessary to provide the patient with an explanation of the procedure, why it is necessary, what alternative diagnostic aid is available, what the risks are, and what effect the lack of high-quality diagnostic films may have on treatment and prognosis. This explanation must be in understandable terms, and the patient must be in full control of his or her senses (e.g., not under the influence of drugs or alcohol). If the patient is a minor, the parent or guardian must be informed about the procedure. The patient's consent may be implied or expressed. When the procedure has risks associated with it, such as from ionizing radiation, receiving expressed consent is strongly recommended. A consent form signed by the patient and dated is the best documentation.

Radiographs are an integral part of the patient's record. The clinician has primary "custodial rights" to the patient's records, but the patient has "property rights," which means the patient has reasonable access to those records. The patient has the right to have the records forwarded to other professionals such as specialists or to a new dentist if the patient moves, to third-party providers, and, possibly, to the courts in litigation procedures. Prudent practice may be to forward diagnostic-quality duplicates of the records, keeping the originals with the patient file.

Study Questions

1. Which of the following PIDs will result in the lowest exposure to a patient, assuming the use of paralleling principles and time-temperature processing?
   A. 16-inch clear rectangular PID.
   B. 8-inch lead-lined cylindrical PID.
   C. 16-inch lead-lined cylindrical PID.
   D. 16-inch rectangular lead-lined PID.
   E. 16-inch clear cylindrical PID.

2. Genetic mutations produced by irradiation of the gonads (reproductive organs) occur
   A. Only when the whole-body dose exceeds 5 rad/yr (0.05 Gy).
   B. Only when the gonad dose exceeds 5 rad/yr (0.05 Gy).
   C. Only when the whole-body dose exceeds the MPD.
   D. Whenever radiation is absorbed by the gonads, regardless of the dose received.

3. The maximum permissible dose for an occupationally exposed worker is
    A. 0.10 Sv/yr (10 rem/yr).
    B. 0.05 Sv/yr (5 rem/yr).
    C. 0.005 Sv/yr (0.5 rem/yr).
    D. 0; no occupational exposure is acceptable.

4. The maximum permissible dose for an occupationally exposed worker who is pregnant is
    A. The same as for a nonpregnant worker.
    B. 0.05 Sv/yr (5 rem/yr).
    C. 0.005 Sv/yr (0.5 rem/yr).
    D. 0; no occupational exposure is acceptable.

5. X radiation affects the incidence of cancer, leukemia, and other abnormalities by
    A. Increasing their incidence among the general population.
    B. Increasing the patient's incidence of each disease.
    C. Producing specific types of cancer or other abnormalities more often.
    D. Storing the radiation within the tissue, creating continual damage after exposure has ceased.

6. Damage to a living organism that is produced by photons striking the organism and producing a molecular chemical change may be caused by
    A. Breaking molecules into smaller pieces.
    B. Disrupting molecular bonds.
    C. Forming new bonds within molecules.
    D. Forming new bonds between molecules.
    E. All of the above.

7. The damaging process in Question 6 is a description of
    A. The somatic effect of radiation absorption.
    B. The direct effect of radiation absorption.
    C. The indirect effect of radiation absorption.
    D. Both direct and indirect effects of radiation absorption.

8. Mutations from radiation exposure can occur
    A. Only in reproductive organs as genetic abnormalities.
    B. In both somatic and reproductive tissue.
    C. Only in the "critical organs."
    D. Only in the cytoplasm.

9. Which of the following is *not* considered a critical organ?
    A. Brain and spinal cord.
    B. Bone marrow.
    C. Gonads.
    D. Thyroid gland.

10. Acute radiation exposure could be described as
    A. Small doses of radiation given over a long period of time, which are less biologically damaging than a chronic exposure of the same amount.
    B. A large dose of radiation given over a very short period of time, which is more biologically damaging than a chronic exposure of the same amount.
    C. Small doses of radiation given over a very short period of time, which are less biologically damaging than a chronic exposure of the same amount.

11. Certain cells and tissues are more sensitive to radiation than others. Which of the following has the lowest sensitivity?
    A. Small lymphocytes and intestinal mucosa.
    B. Nerve and muscle.
    C. Bone marrow.
    D. Reproductive cells.
    E. Skin and oral mucosa.

12. Which of the following is not a good way to reduce exposure?
    A. Using fast film; "E" speed is the fastest.
    B. Using an 8-inch PID.
    C. Using the paralleling technique.
    D. Using higher kilovoltage settings.
    E. Using a rectangular lead-lined PID.

13. It is important to obtain informed consent from the patient before exposing him or her to ionizing radiation. Which of the following is not a necessary part of the "informed consent" receiving process?
    A. Explaining what will be done in the procedure.
    B. Explaining why the procedure is necessary.
    C. Explaining what the risks are.
    D. Explaining what alternatives are available.
    E. Giving the patient a copy of the radiograph schedule (i.e., scheduling bitewings once a year, a CMRS every 5 years).

14. The 1981 Consumer-Patient Radiation Health and Safety Act addresses the legal responsibility for
    A. Quality and maintenance of equipment.
    B. Accreditation of personnel training programs.
    C. Inspection of equipment.
    D. Mandatory certification of all operators of ionizing radiation equipment.
    E. All of the above.

Glossary of Radiologic Terms*

Absorb To take into the skin or body tissue.

Absorbed Dose *See* Dose.

Absorption A process whereby the intensity of a beam of radiation is reduced because some (or all) of the particles (or photons) of the incident beam are eliminated or reduced in energy by interactions with matter.

Accelerator, Developer *See* Developer

Acid A solution containing more hydrogen ions than water. Its pH is less than 7. The hydrogen ions can be replaced by a base to form salts.

Actinic Radiation Radiation that can produce photochemical effects, such as the production of a latent image in a film emulsion by visible light or x-rays.

Actual Focal Spot The area of the target (tungsten) that is always larger than the effective focal size. It is the area of the anode upon which the electrons strike. *See also* Effective Focal Spot

Acute Exposure Radiation exposure of short duration; usually refers to radiation of relatively high intensity.

Adaptation (Dark) The adaptation of the eye in the dark.

Age Fog Fogging, either mottled or uniform, owing to outdated film or films stored under conditions of excessively high temperature and humidity.

Alternating Current A flow of electrons in one direction followed by a flow in the opposite direction.

Aluminum Filter Any of various thicknesses of aluminum used as filtration in an x-ray beam to absorb the longer-wavelength, less-penetrating radiation.

Ammonium Thiosulfate. *See* Fixer

Ampere The unit of intensity of an electric current produced by 1 volt acting through a resistance of 1 ohm.

Anatomic Landmark An anatomic structure that serves as an aid in the localization and identification of regions to be radiographed.

Angulation The direction of the primary beam of radiation in relation to object and film. There is a horizontal and vertical angulation to the beam.

Anion An ion carrying a negative charge.

Anode The positive terminal of an x-ray tube; a tungsten block embedded in a copper stem and set at an angle to the cathode *(q.v.)*. The anode emits x rays from the point of impact of the electron stream from the cathode. A *rotating anode* is one that rotates constantly during x-ray production to present a changing focal spot to the electron stream and to permit use of smaller focal spots or higher tube voltages or currents without overheating.

Anteroposterior Position (AP) An examination in which the film is placed at the posterior location (for example, the back of the head), with the x rays passing from the anterior to the posterior direction.

AP *See* Anteroposterior Position (AP)

Area Monitoring Routine monitoring of the level of radiation in any particular area, building, room, or equipment.

Artifact Either (1) a substance or structure not naturally present in living tissues but that produces an authentic image in a radiograph; or (2) a blemish or unintended radiographic image resulting from faulty manufacture, manipulation, exposure, or processing of an x-ray film.

Atom The smallest part of an element that is capable of entering into a chemical

---

*Adapted from Schiff T, Nummikoski P: Glossary of Maxillofacial Radiology, 3rd ed., American Academy of Oral and Maxillofacial Radiology, Jackson, MS, 1990.

reaction. It consists of a positively charged nucleus and an extranuclear portion composed of electrons equal in number to the nuclear protons.

Atomic Number   The number of electrons outside the nucleus of a neutral atom. It is also the number of protons in the nucleus.

Background (Radiation)   Background implies radioactivity arising from nature. This includes cosmic rays *(q.v.)* and radioactive elements in the earth and air.

Backscatter   Radiation deflected by scattering processes at angles greater than 90 degrees to the original direction of the beam of radiation. *See also* Scattered Radiation

Barrier, Protective   A barrier of radiation-absorbing material, such as lead, concrete, or plaster, used to reduce radiation hazards. A *primary protective barrier* is a barrier sufficient to reduce the useful beam to the permissible dose rate. A *secondary protective barrier* is a barrier sufficient to reduce the secondary, or scatter, radiation to the permissible dose rate.

Base   A solution containing fewer hydrogen ions than water. Its pH is greater than 7. Bases can react with acids to form salts.

Beam   An emission of electromagnetic radiation or particles. A *central beam* is the center of the beam of x rays emitted from an x-ray tube, usually called the *central ray*. A *useful beam* is the part of the primary radiation that is permitted to emerge from the tubehead assembly of an x-ray machine, as limited by the tubehead port and accessory collimating devices.

Beam-Guiding Instrument   Instrument used during radiography to facilitate correct alignment of the central ray. *See also* Position-Indicating Device (PID)

BEIR Committee   Advisory committee on the biological effects of ionizing radiation.

Binding Energy   The energy needed to eject an electron from the atom.

Bisecting-angle Technique   A technique for the radiographic exposure of intraoral films whereby the central axis or central ray of the x-ray beam is directed at right angles to a plane determined by bisecting the angle formed by (1) the long axis of the tooth or teeth being radiographed and (2) the plane in which the film is positioned behind the teeth.

Bitewing Radiograph   The x-ray shadow images of the crowns, necks, and coronal thirds of the roots of both upper and lower teeth, so called because the patient bites on a cardboard tab, or "wing," placed in the center of the film packet.

Block   In intraoral radiography a block is a film holder that the patient bites on to provide stable retention of the film packet or orientation of tooth position. In panoramic radiography a block is a tooth positioner that provides correct orientation of the dentition within the image layer.

"Boiling Off" Electrons   Heat or incandescence of the filament of the x-ray tube, which produces a source of free electrons by thermionic emission.

Bound Electron   An electron that is close to the nucleus: for example, the K shell electron.

Bremsstrahlung Radiation   A spectral distribution of x rays ranging from very low-energy photons to those produced by the peak kilovoltage applied across an x-ray tube. Bremsstrahlung means "braking radiation," referring to the sudden deceleration of electrons as they interact with highly positively charged nuclei.

Calcium Tungstate   A chemical substance in crystal form used to coat radiographic intensifying screens; the screens fluoresce when struck by x rays.

Carcinogen   A substance having the ability to produce cancer.

Cassette A light-tight container in which x-ray films are placed for exposure to x radiation; usually backed with lead to reduce the effect of backscattered radiation *(q.v.)*. A *screen-type cassette* is a film holder, usually made of metal, with the exposure side made of a low-atomic-number material such as Bakelite, aluminum, or magnesium; the cassette contains intensifying screens between which a "screen type" film is placed for exposure.

Cathode A negative electrode from which electrons are emitted. In x-ray tubes, the cathode usually consists of a helical tungsten filament behind which a molybdenum reflector cup is located to focus the electron emission toward the target of the anode.

Cathode Ray A stream of electrons passing from the hot filament of the cathode to the target, or anode, in an x-ray tube.

Cathode Ray Tube A tube cathode containing a spirally wound filament that becomes incandescent, producing electrons when a low-voltage electric current is passed through it.

Cation A positively charged ion.

Cell A minute protoplasmic mass that in the aggregate makes up organized tissue. The cell consists of a circumscribed mass that contains a nucleus and a surrounding cytoplasm. *Germ cells* have the function of reproducing an entity similar to the organism from which the germ cells originate. They are characteristically haploid, i.e., have a single set of chromosomes. *Somatic cells* are body cells (any cells that are not germ cells); they are characteristically diploid, i.e., have two sets of chromosomes.

Centigrade (C°) The metric temperature scale on which the freezing point of water is 0 and the boiling point of water is 100. The formula for the conversion of degrees centigrade to degrees Fahrenheit is $F° = 9/5 \, C° + 32$.

Central Ray The theoretical center of the x-ray beam. The term is employed to designate the direction of the x rays in a given projection; the central ray may be considered to extend from the focal spot of the x-ray tube to the x-ray film.

Cephalometric Projection Examination by means of film placed to obtain lateral and Caldwell posteroanterior views of the head. Used in orthodontics, maxillofacial surgery, and, to some degree, in prosthodontics to measure and study maxillofacial growth and maxillary and mandibular relationships. The head is held in position by means of a holding device called a cephalostat.

Cervical Pertaining to (1) the neck, or cervical vertebrae, and (2) the cementoenamel junction (CEJ) area of a tooth.

Characteristic (Discrete) Radiation Electromagnetic radiation produced by electron transitions from higher energy orbitals to replace ejected electrons of inner electron orbitals. The energy of the electromagnetic radiation emitted is unique to and characteristic of the emitting atom (element).

Chromosome Aberration Any rearrangement of chromosome parts as a result of breakage by radiation or other means.

Chronic Exposure Radiation exposure of long duration, either continuous (protracted exposure) or intermittent (fractionation exposure); usually refers to exposure of relatively low intensity.

Clearing Agent. Agent in the fixer used to remove nonactivated silver halide crystals.

Coherent Scattering Sometimes called *unmodified scattering*. One of the four interactions that occur when photons (x rays) and atoms collide with each other. The low-energy x-ray photon collides with an inner-orbital electron, but its low energy cannot dislodge the electron. The electron may absorb the photon, which then sets the photon into vibration. This causes an electromagnetic wave that is the same as the incident (incoming) photon but that travels in a different direction. This type of interaction is below the energy range useful in clinical radiology.

Collimation   Any device used for the elimination of the peripheral divergent portion of the useful x-ray beam, such as metal tubes, "cones," or diaphragms interposed in the path of the beam.

Collimator   A lead disc with an aperture of various sizes and shapes. The diaphragm limits the size of the primary beam to the area of interest, thereby minimizing patient exposure to the primary beam.

Compton Scatter Radiation   Commonly called *scatter radiation*. The incident radiation has sufficient energy to dislodge a bound electron; when it attacks a loosely bound electron and dislodges it, the remaining radiation energy proceeds in a different direction as scatter radiation.

Condyle   A rounded projection on a bone, usually for articulation with another bone (e.g., of the mandible).

Cone   A device on a dental x-ray machine that is designed to indicate the direction of the central ray and to serve as a guide in establishing a desired source-to-film distance (SFD). A *short cone* establishes an anode-to-skin distance of up to approximately 18 cm. A *long cone* establishes an extended anode-to-skin distance, usually within the range of 27 cm to 36 cm.

Cone Cutting   Failure to cover or expose the entire area of a radiograph with the useful beam, thereby only partially exposing the film.

Cone Distance   The distance between the focal spot and the end of the cone, usually expressed in inches or centimeters.

Constant Potential Kilovoltage.   *See* Kilovoltage

Continuous Spectrum   For electromagnetic radiation, a spectrum that exhibits a gradual variation of wavelength. Examples include the spectrum of light from an incandescent solid and an x-ray spectrum.

Contrast   The difference in image density appearing on a radiograph, representing various degrees of beam attenuation.

>   *Film contrast:*   A characteristic inherent in the type of film used.

>   *Long-scale contrast:*   An increased range of grays between the blacks and whites on a radiograph. Higher kilovoltages increase this range.

>   *Short-scale contrast:*   A reduced range of grays between the blacks and whites on a radiograph. Lower kilovoltages decrease this range.

>   *Subject contrast:*   The relative difference in density and thickness of the components of the radiographed subject, as evidenced by the varied radiographic densities caused by the difference in absorbing power of the different kinds of material traversed by an x-ray beam.

Cosmic Rays   Radiation of extremely short wavelengths that originates outside the earth's atmosphere.

Critical Tissues (Organs)   Those tissues that either react unfavorably to radiation or, by their nature, attract and absorb specific radiochemicals.

Crookes' Tube   *See* X-ray Tube

Darkroom   A room that can be completely darkened so that photographic or x-ray film may be processed.

Daylight System   A method of loading, unloading, and feeding films into the processor in normal room light. This system entails the use of special equipment, with no need for a darkroom.

Definition (Image) The property of images pertaining to their sharpness, distinctness, or clarity.

Density (Photographic or Film) The degree of darkening of exposed and processed photographic or x-ray film.

Background density: The density of a processed film owing to factors other than the radiation exposure received through the recorded objects or structures.

Inherent (film) density: The density of a processed film owing to such intrinsic factors in the film as the density of the film base and the emulsion gelatin.

Object (tissue) density: The resistance of an object to the passage of x rays.

Detail A visual quality that depends on sharpness (definition). Factors that influence detail include (1) the size of the tube focal spot, (2) the source-to-film distance, (3) the distance of the object from the film, (4) the motion of the object or x-ray source, (5) the type of intensifying screens, and (6) the image contrast.

Developer A chemical (potassium bromide) used in a developer to check the development of the unexposed silver bromide and to control the working speed of the developer with respect to the exposed silver bromide. The developer also contains a reducing agent.

Directly Ionizing Particles Charged particles having sufficient kinetic energy to produce ionization by collision.

Distal Remote; farther from any point of reference; e.g., midline.

Distortion An inaccuracy in the size or shape of an object as it is displayed in the radiograph. *Magnification distortion* is the proportional enlargement of a radiographic image. It is always present to some degree in oral radiography but is minimized with increased source-to-film distance or decreased object-to-film distance. *Vertical distortion* is the disproportional change in size, either elongation or foreshortening owing to incorrect vertical angulation or improper film placement.

Dose (Dosage of Radiation) The amount of energy absorbed per unit mass of tissue at a site of interest.

Absorbed dose: The amount of energy imparted by ionizing radiation to a unit mass of irradiated material at a place of interest. The unit of absorbed dose in the traditional system is the *rad* (100 ergs/g). The currently accepted unit of absorbed dose is the *gray* (Gy). (1 Gy = 1 joule/kg.)

Cumulative dose: The total dose resulting from repeated exposures to radiation of the same region, or of the whole body.

Depth dose: The radiation delivered to a particular depth beneath the surface of the body; it is usually expressed as a percentage of surface dose.

Doubling dose: The amount of ionizing radiation absorbed by the gonads of the average person in a population over a period of several generations that will result in a doubling of the current rate of spontaneous mutations.

Erythema dose: Antiquated measurement based on the amount of radiation that will cause erythema (redness) of the skin.

Exit dose: The absorbed dose delivered by a beam of radiation to the surface through which the beam emerges from an object.

Threshold dose: The minimum dose that will produce a detectable degree of any given effect.

Tissue dose: The radiation dose received by a tissue. In the case of x rays and gamma rays, tissue doses are expressed in *rads*. The *rem* is the generally accepted unit of tissue dose for other ionizing radiations.

Dose Equivalent The product of absorbed dose and modifying factors (i.e., the quality factor, distribution factor, and any other necessary factors). The traditional unit of dose equivalence is the *rem* (rad × qualifying factors). The international system (SI) unit of dose equivalence is the sievert (Sv) (grays × qualifying factors).

Dosimeter (Radiation Meter) An instrument used to detect and measure an accumulated dosage of radiation.

Double Exposure Two superimposed exposures on the same radiographic or photographic film.

Effective Focal Spot The apparent size and shape of the focal spot when viewed from a position in the useful beam; with the use of a suitable inclined anode face, it is smaller than the actual focal spot size. *See also* Line Focus

Ektaspeed Film Direct-exposure film with a speed *(q.v.)* category of approximately 25 R^{-1}.

Electrode Either of the two terminals of an electric source, an anode or a cathode *(q.q.v.)*.

Electromagnetic Radiation The forms of energy propagated by wave motion as photons or discrete quanta. The radiations have no matter associated with them. They differ widely in wavelength, frequency, and photon energy and have strikingly different properties. Covering an enormous range of wavelengths (from 10^{17} to 10^{-6} angstroms), they include radio waves, infrared waves, visible light, ultraviolet radiation, x rays, gamma rays, and cosmic radiation.

Electromagnetic Wave A wave produced by mutual induction of electric and magnetic fields.

Electron A negatively charged elementary particle.

Electron Stream Electrons moving from the cathode to the anode across a potential difference in a low-pressure gas tube or a vacuum tube.

Electron Volt The kinetic energy gained by an electron falling through a potential difference of 1 volt.

Element A pure substance consisting of atoms of the same atomic number, which cannot be decomposed by ordinary chemical means.

Elon. *See* Developer

Elongation A form of radiographic distortion in which the image is longer than the object radiographed.

Entrance Dose Dose measured at the surface of an irradiated object. It includes both primary radiation and backscatter from the irradiated underlying material.

Epithelium The cells lining all canals and body surfaces, including those cells that are specialized for secretion.

Equivalent The thickness of pure aluminum, concrete, or lead that would afford the same radiation attenuation, under specified conditions, as any given material being considered.

Excitation The addition of energy to a system, thereby transferring it from its ground state to an excited state.

Exit Dose. *See* Dose

Exposure A measure of the ionization produced in air by x radiation or gamma radiation. It is the sum of the electrical charges on all of the ions of one sign produced in air when all of the electrons liberated by the photons in a volume element of air are completely stopped in air, divided by the mass of the air in the volume element.

Exposure Factors   Radiographic kilovoltage, exposure time, milliamperage, and source-to-film distance: the primary radiographic factors considered when making an exposure.

External Oblique Ridge   A ridge originating from the anterior border of the ramus of the mandible extending to the lateral body of the mandible in the molar region.

Extraoral Radiograph   An examination of the teeth and bones made by placing the film or cassette against the side of the head or face and projecting the x rays from the opposite side.

Filament   A coiled tungsten wire that emits electrons when heated to incandescence.

Film   A thin, transparent sheet of cellulose acetate or similar material coated on one or both sides with an emulsion sensitive to radiation and light. *Direct-exposure film* is highly sensitive to the direct action of x rays but has low sensitivity to screen fluorescence (e.g., intraoral dental film). *Screen film* is sensitive to the fluorescent light of intensifying screens but not as sensitive to the direct action of x rays (e.g., panoramic film). *X-ray film* is (1) film manufactured for use in radiography or (2) a radiograph.

Film Badge   A metal container of radiographic film used for the detection and measurement of radiation exposure of personnel.

Film Base   The thin, transparent sheet of cellulose acetate or similar material that carries the radiation- and light-sensitive emulsion of x-ray films.

Film Packet   A lightproof, moisture-resistant, sealed paper or plastic envelope containing x-ray film, used in making radiographs.

Film Processing   The process of converting a latent image to a visible image by immersion in developer and fixer, followed by rinsing in water and drying.

Film Speed   The amount of exposure to light or x rays (the latter in roentgens) required to produce a given image density. Film speed is expressed as the reciprocal of the exposure in roentgens necessary to produce a density of 1.0 above base and fog. Films are classified on the basis in six speed groups, from A through F. *See* Speed

Filter   The material (usually aluminum) placed in the useful beam to absorb preferentially the less energetic (less penetrating) radiations.

Filtration   The use of absorbers or filters for the preferential attenuation of radiation of certain wavelengths from a useful primary beam of x radiation.

Fixation.   *See* Fixer

Fixer (Film or Hypo-)   The solution (primarily ammonium thiosulfate) in which the manifest image is fixed and hardened, removing the silver halide crystals from the exposed film that was unexposed to or unaffected by the action of the x radiation.

Fluorescence   The emission of radiation of a particular wavelength by certain substances as the result of absorption of radiation of shorter wavelength. The emission occurs essentially only during the period of irradiation.

Fluorescent Screen   A sheet of material coated with a substance, e.g., calcium tungstate or zinc sulfide, that emits visible light when irradiated with x radiation.

Focal Spot   The part of the target on the anode of an x-ray tube that is bombarded by the focused electron stream when the tube is energized.

Focusing Cup   Along with the filament, the focusing cup determines the size and shape of the target (focal) spot. The cup is constructed of molybdenum.

Fog (Fogging)   A darkening of the whole or part of a radiograph by sources other than the radiation of the primary beam to which the film was exposed. *Chemical fog* is film darkening owing to imbalance or deterioration of processing solutions. *Light fog* is darkening owing to unintentional exposure to light (to which the emulsion is sensitive), either before or during processing. *Radiation fog* is darkening owing to radiation from sources other than intentional exposure to the primary beam (e.g., scatter radiation), or exposure of film during unprotected storage.

Foreshortening   A form of distortion in which the image is shorter than the object radiographed. In the angle-bisecting technique it is caused by misdirecting the x-ray beam perpendicular to the plane of the film instead of to the plane of the bisector (i.e., the vertical angulation is too steep).

Gadolinium and Lanthanum   Phosphors that absorb more of the available x-ray photons and have a higher conversion efficiency to light than does calcium tungstate, the phosphor most commonly used in intensifying screens. Sometimes referred to as *rare-earth elements*.

Gamma Radiation   Short-wavelength electromagnetic radiation of nuclear origin, within a range of wavelengths from about 10^{-8} cm to 10^{-11} cm.

Gelatin   A protein obtained from animal skin and hooves by boiling; used in x-ray film manufacture as a means of suspending the silver halide crystals in the film emulsion.

Gene   The fundamental unit of inheritance that determines and controls transmissible characteristics.

Genetic Effects (Radiation)   Changes produced in the genes and chromosomes of all nucleated body cells. In customary usage, the term relates to the effect produced in the reproductive cells.

Geometric Unsharpness   Impairment of image definition owing to the penumbra (shadow).

Gonad   An ovary or a testis; the site of origin of oocytes or spermatozoa.

Gray   A unit of radiation measurement established in 1974 by the International Commission on Radiation Units and Measurements. One gray (Gy) = 1 joule/kg = 100 rad. The gray is a unit of absorbed dose and replaces the rad.

Grid   A device used to prevent as much scattered radiation as possible from reaching an x-ray film during the exposure of a radiograph.

H and D Curve   A characteristic curve of a photographic emulsion obtained by plotting film density against the logarithm of the exposure. Also called the *Hurter and Driffield curve* (named after the British scientists and founders).

Halides   Compounds of metals with halogen elements: bromine, chlorine, and iodine.

"Hard" Radiation   A slang term for x rays of short wavelengths and high penetrating power. In usage, the shorter the wavelength is, the "harder" the radiation.

Horizontal Angulation.   *See* Angulation

Impulse   The burst of radiation generated during a half-cycle of alternating current.

Indirectly Ionizing Particles   Uncharged particles that can liberate directly ionizing particles or can initiate a nuclear transformation.

Interpretation (of X-Ray Film)   The study of a radiograph, the interpretation of that which is seen, and the integration of the findings with the case history, laboratory, and clinical examinations to arrive at a diagnosis.

Interproximal (Bitewing) Radiograph   A special type of intraoral radiograph for depicting interproximal features of the teeth and interdental bone crests, made on a film positioned by special (bitewing) tabs on which the patient's teeth are closed.

Intraoral Radiograph Radiograph produced on a film placed intraorally to the teeth.

Inverse Square Law of Radiation The intensity or exposure rate of radiation at a given distance from the source is inversely proportional to the square of the distance.

Ion An atomic particle, atom, or chemical radical bearing an electrical charge, either negative or positive.

Ionization The process or the result of a process by which a neutral atom or molecule acquires either a positive or a negative charge.

Ionizing Radiation Electromagnetic radiation (x rays or gamma rays) or particulate radiation (electrons, neutrons, and protons) capable of ionizing air directly or indirectly.

K Electron An electron having an orbit in the K shell, which is the first shell of electrons surrounding the atom's nucleus.

keV The symbol for 1,000 electron volts.

Kilo (k) A prefix representing 1,000.

Kilovoltage (in x-ray machines) The potential difference between the anode and the cathode of an x-ray tube. *Constant-potential kilovoltage* is the potential formed by a constant-voltage generator expressed as constant-potential kilovolts (kVcp).

Kilovoltage Peak (kVp) The crest value (in kilovolts) of the potential difference of a pulsating-potential generator. When only half of the wave is used, the value refers to the useful half of the cycle.

Lamina Dura The thin plate of dense, or compact, bone that lines the tooth sockets; it appears on a radiograph as a fine radiopaque line passing around the tooth.

Latent Image The invisible change produced in a photographic or x-ray film emulsion by the action of x radiation or light, from which the visible image is subsequently developed and fixed chemically.

Latent Period The period between the time of exposure of tissue to an injurious agent (i.e., radiation) and the clinical manifestation of a particular response.

Lateral Jaw Projection An examination in which the film is placed adjacent to the patient's ramus, or the body of the mandible, with the rays directed obliquely upward from the opposite side and the central beam directed at the point of interest. The vertical angulation is such that it casts the image of the near mandible superior or anterior to the area of interest.

Lateral Skull Projection An examination in which the film is placed parallel to the sagittal plane of the patient's head with the rays directed at right angles to the plane of the film and the sagittal plane; the entire skull is shown.

Latitude, Film Exposure The range between the minimum and maximum radiation exposures that yields diagnostically useful images of structures.

Latitude, Object The range between the maximum and minimum object densities recorded on a radiograph.

Leaded Apron A lead-impregnated rubber apron that provides protection for patients and auxiliary personnel from radiation.

Leukemia A disease in which there is great overproduction of white blood cells, or a relative overproduction of immature white cells, and great enlargement of the spleen. It can result from exposure to ionizing radiation.

Line Focus   A principle employed in the design of x-ray tubes, by which the effective focal spot *(q.v.)* is sharply reduced relative to the actual focal spot.

Localization   The making of a radiograph for the purpose of identifying a site in relation to surrounding tissues.

Long Cone.   *See* Cone

Long-Scale Contrast.   *See* Contrast

mA.   *See* Milliampere (mA)

mAs.   *See* Milliampere-Seconds (mAs)

Magnification, Radiographic   The enlargement or distortion of a radiographic image recorded on film emulsion, minimized by reducing the object-to-film distance and increasing the focal-film distance.

Magnification Distortion.   *See* Distortion

Maximum Permissible Dose (MPD)   The MPD is the maximum dose of radiation that, in view of present knowledge, is not expected to produce significant radiation effects. For radiation workers, 50 mSv per year is permissible.

Mesial   Toward the center of the dental arch.

Milliampere (mA)   Electrically, the milliampere is 1/1,000 of an ampere *(q.v.)*. In radiography, milliamperage refers to the current flow from the cathode to the anode, which in turn regulates the intensity of radiation emitted by the x-ray tube and hence directly influences the radiographic density.

Milliampere-Seconds (mAs)   The product of the x-ray tube operating amperage and exposure time in seconds.

Millimeter (mm)   One-thousandth of a meter.

Millirad (mrad)   One-thousandth of a rad.

Millirem (mrem)   One-thousandth of a rem.

Milliroentgen (mR)   One-thousandth of a roentgen.

Molecule   The smallest quantity of matter that can exist by itself and retain its chemical properties; it is composed of one or more atoms.

Monochromatic Radiation   Electromagnetic radiation of a single wavelength.

Mutation   A departure from the parent type, as when an organism differs from its parents in one or more heritable characteristics as a result of genetic change.

Neutron   An elementary particle having no electrical charge. The neutron is a constituent of the nucleus of all atoms except hydrogen.

Nucleus, Atomic   The small central part of an atom containing the protons and neutrons; most of the atomic mass is concentrated here.

Object Density.   *See* Density

Object-to-Film Distance (OFD)   Distance between the object or skin and the cassette or film.

Oblique   An angular view of a surface or object.

Occlusal Plane   The plane of the masticating surfaces of the molar and bicuspid teeth when the maxilla and mandible are closed.

Occlusal Radiograph   A radiograph made with a film designed for placement between the occlusal surfaces of the teeth, with the x-ray beam directed caudad or cephalad.

Orbital Electron   An electron that is moving in an orbit around the nucleus of an atom.

Osteoradionecrosis   Damage and death of normal bone that may result from a curative dose of radiation used in the treatment of malignant or nonmalignant disease.

Overdevelopment   Permitting the film to remain in the developer beyond the normal or preset time. This decreases radiographic contrast and increases radiographic density.

Oxidation   A chemical reaction in which an electron is removed from an atom.

Panoramic Radiograph.   *See* Pantomography

Pantomography   A method of radiography by which continuous radiographs of the maxillary or mandibular dental arches and their associated structures may be obtained.

Paralleling (Right-Angle) Technique   The production of a radiographic exposure of intraoral film whereby the plane of the film packet is made parallel to the long axis of the tooth being radiographed. The central beam axis, or "central ray" of the x ray, is directed at right angles to both.

Peak Kilovoltage.   *See* Kilovoltage Peak

Penetrability   The ability of a beam of x radiation to pass through matter; kilovoltage and filtration determine the degree of penetrability.

Penumbra   The secondary shadow that surrounds the periphery of the primary shadow; the term pertains to the shadow proper. A penumbra is the ill-defined margin or shadow produced by light. In radiography it is the blurred margin of an image detail, also called *geometric unsharpness.*

Periapical Radiograph   A radiograph made by intraoral placement of film for recording shadow images of the outline, position, and mesiodistal extent of the teeth and surrounding tissue.

Photoelectric Effect   The ejection of bound electrons by an incident photon such that the whole energy of the photon is absorbed and transitional or characteristic x-ray emissions are produced.

Photoelectron   An electron emitted from a substance under a stimulus or other radiation of appropriate wavelength. *See* Photoelectric Effect

Photon   A quantum of electromagnetic radiation.

PID.   *See* Position-Indicating Device (PID)

Position-Indicating Device (PID)   A device usually composed of a plastic ring through which a metal rod can be placed to assist in properly aligning the cone and film (see Chapter 1).

Potassium Bromide.   *See* Developer

Preservative   A chemical that inhibits oxidation of the reducing agents by air. Sodium sulfite is the chemical usually employed as a preservative.

Projection   A term for the position of a part of the patient's anatomy with relation to the x-ray film and the x-ray beam.

Protective Barrier   A barrier of radiation-absorbing material(s) used to reduce radiation exposure. *The primary protective barrier* is a barrier sufficient to attenuate the useful beam to the required degree. The *secondary protective barrier* is a barrier sufficient to attenuate the scatter, or secondary radiation, to the required degree.

Proton   An elementary nuclear particle with a positive electric charge.

Proximal   Nearest: closest to a point of reference.

Quality Assurance   Maintaining continuously optimal functioning of both technical and operational aspects of radiologic procedures—to produce maximal diagnostic information while minimizing patient exposure to radiation.

Quality Factor (QF)   The linear-energy-transfer-dependent factor by which absorbed doses are multiplied to obtain (for radiation protection purposes) a quantity that expresses the effect of the absorbed dose on a common scale for all ionizing radiations.

Rad (Radiation-Absorbed Dose; Roentgen-Absorbed Dose)   A unit of measurement for the absorbed dose of any type of ionizing radiation in any medium. One rad is the energy absorption of 100 ergs (*cf.* Gray).

Radiation   The emission and propagation of energy in the form of waves or particles through space or a material medium. *See also* Magnification, Radiographic; Monochromatic Radiation

Radiation, Actinic   Radiation that can produce photochemical effects, such as the production of a latent image in a film emulsion by visible light or x rays.

Radiation Burn   A burn caused by overexposure to radiant energy.

Radiation Dermatitis   Inflammation of the skin resulting from a high dose of radiation. The reaction varies with the quality and quantity of radiation used and is usually transitory.

Radiation Sickness   A syndrome associated with exposure to ionizing radiation that may result in nausea, vomiting, and diarrhea; later symptoms include malaise, depression, epilation, purpura, hemorrhage, fever, and emaciation.

Radiobiology   That branch of biology dealing with radiation effects on biologic systems.

Radiograph   A visible image on a radiation-sensitive film emulsion produced by chemical processing after exposure of the film emulsion to ionizing radiation that has passed through an area, region, or substance of interest.

Radiographic Survey   A series of radiographic projections constituting a study.

Radiography   The technical process of positioning, exposing, and processing radiographs.

Radiologic Health   The art and science of protecting humans from injury by radiation, as well as of promoting better health through beneficial applications of radiation.

Radiolucency   The appearance of dark images on film owing to the greater amount of radiation that penetrates the structures and reaches the film.

Radiolucent   Permitting the passage of x rays with relatively little attenuation by absorption.

Radiopacity   The appearance of light images on film owing to the lesser amount of radiation that penetrates the structures and reaches the film.

Radiopaque   Strongly inhibiting the passage of x rays.

Radiosensitivity   Relative susceptibility of cells, tissues, organs, organisms, or any substances to the injurious action of radiation.

Rare Earth   Commonly used to refer to intensifying screens that contain one or more of the rare-earth elements and that use the absorption and conversion features of these elements in x-ray imaging. May also refer to a screen-film system used for x-ray imaging. These systems are considered "fast" exposure systems.

RBE (Relative Biological Effectiveness)   A factor used to compare the biologic effects of absorbed dosages of differing types of ionizing radiation in a particular organism or tissue. The standard of comparison is medium-voltage x rays delivered at about 10 rads per minute. The unit of RBE is the *rem (q.v.).*

Rectification   Conversion of alternating current to direct current. *Full-wave rectification* is conversion of the entire wave of an alternating current to a direct current. *Half-wave rectification* is conversion of half of the sine wave of an alternating current to a direct current. *Self-rectification* is rectification of half of the sine wave of the alternating current across an x-ray tube as a result of the absence of electron emission at the anode.

Reducing Agent. *See* Developer

Relative Risk   The ratio of the risk of biologic harm: in those exposed, to the risk; in those not exposed, to radiation.

Rem (Roentgen-Equivalent-Man)   A unit of dose of any radiation to body tissue, expressed in terms of its estimated biologic effects relative to an exposure of 1 roentgen of gamma or x radiation.

Resolution (Image)   The discernible separation of closely adjacent image details. In optics, to separate and make visible the parts of an image.

Reticulation   A network of corrugations in the emulsion of a radiograph as a result of too great a difference in temperature between any two of the three darkroom solutions.

Roentgen (R)   An international unit of exposure based on the ability of radiation to ionize air; an exposure to gamma or x radiation such that the associated corpuscular emission per 0.0001293 gram of air produces, in air, ions carrying 1 electrostatic unit of quantity of either positive or negative electricity (2.083 billion ion pairs).

Roentgen, Wilhelm C. (German spelling: Röntgen)   The discoverer of x rays; on November 8, 1895, he observed that a Crookes' vacuum tube operating at high voltage caused a piece of barium platinocyanide lying a few feet away from the tube to glow in the dark. Dr. Roentgen, a physicist, is known as the "father of x rays."

Safelight   Special lighting used in the darkroom that permits film to be transferred from cassette to processor without fogging.

Scattered Radiation   Radiation that, during passage through a substance, has been deviated in direction. It may also have been modified by an increase in wavelengths. Scattered radiation is one form of secondary radiation *(q.v.)*.

Secondary Ionization   Particles, usually electrons, ejected by recoil when a primary ionizing particle passes through matter.

Secondary Radiation   Particles or photons produced by the interaction of primary radiation with matter.

Sharpness (Image)   The ability of an image to demonstrate an interface line as one-dimensional.

"Soft" Radiation   X rays of relatively long wavelength with relatively little penetrating ability.

Source   The point of emanation of gamma or x rays when used as an origin of radiation.

Spatial Resolution   The smallest distance between two points in an object that can be distinguished as separate detail in the image; generally indicated as a number of black and white line-pairs per millimeter.

Speed, Film   Speed in radiography refers to the relative amount of darkening produced on a film (with reference to film or screen characteristics) from a given amount of radiation. Speed and sensitivity may be used interchangeably. Officially, the speed of a film system is defined as the reciprocal of the exposure in roentgens required to produce a density of 1.0 above base-plus-fog density. The measurement unit of film speed is R^{-1}.

$$\text{speed} = \frac{1}{\text{roentgens (R)}}$$

Speed of Light Light travels 186,000 miles per second. All electromagnetic radiation travels at the speed of light.

Speed of X rays X rays travel at the speed of light, 186,000 miles per second, or at 3×10^8 meters per second in a vacuum.

Static Marks Marks on a radiograph resembling small streaks of lightning; they result from static electricity that occurs when the film is removed from the wrapper paper or when films are separated after being piled on top of one another.

Step-Down Transformer This transformer produces a lower voltage output by stepping down the input voltage. Stepping down the voltage results in a step up in amperage, because the power input is equal to the power output. The filament transformer of the x-ray circuit is a step-down transformer.

Step-Up Transformer This transformer produces a higher voltage output than the input by stepping up the output voltage. Stepping up the voltage results in a step down in amperage, because the power input is equal to the power output. The high-voltage transformer of the x-ray circuit is a step-up transformer.

Stop Bath A solution of water and acetic acid used between the developer and the fixer that stops the development of the film.

Tank, Processing Metal tanks used to hold processing solutions. These tanks are constructed of stainless steel to resist corrosion and permit rapid equalization of temperature control. The outside walls of the tanks are insulated to prevent condensation of moisture and maintain temperature control.

Target The area on the anode subject to electron bombardment, usually consisting of a tungsten insert on the end face of a solid copper anode.

Target-Film Distance (TFD) This is the same as focal-film distance (FFD), in that it is the distance from the focal spot of the x-ray tube to the x-ray film.

Thermionic Emission The release of electrons from the cathode filament by heating.

Timer A switch mechanism used to complete the electrical circuit to produce x rays for a predetermined time. An *electronic timer* is a timer that functions through a mechanical clock mechanism. A *hand timer* is an attachment to or part of a timer that requires thumb or finger pressure to actuate the timing device. A *mechanical timer* is a timer operated by a spring mechanism.

Tissue An aggregation of similarly specialized cells united in the performance of a particular function.

Tumor Either (1) a swelling or a morbid enlargement of tissue or (2) a neoplasm; that is, a mass of new tissue that persists and grows independently of its surrounding structure and that has no physiologic function.

Ultraspeed Film Direct-exposure film with a speed category of approximately 15 R^{-1}.

Umbra A complete shadow produced by light, with sharply demarcated margins. In radiography, a sharply delineated image detail.

Underexposed A condition of a radiograph in which the image displays insufficient silver deposits.

Vertical Angulation *See* Angulation

Volt The unit of electrical pressure or electromotive force necessary to produce a current of 1 ampere through a resistance of 1 ohm. An *electric volt* is the kinetic energy gained by an electron in falling through a potential difference of 1 volt: 1.6×10^{-12} ergs.

Wave, Electromagnetic   Energy manifested by movements in an advancing series of alternating elevations and depressions.

Wavelength   The distance between the peaks of waves in any waveform, such as light, x rays, and other electromotive forms; also the distance from any point on a wave to the identical point on an adjacent wave. In electromagnetic radiation, the wavelength is equal to the velocity of light divided by the frequency of the wave.

Wetting Agent   A solution used in film processing; it follows the washing process to accelerate the flow of water from both film surfaces and to hasten the drying of radiographs.

Whole-Body Radiation   Exposure of the patient's entire body to radiation.

X Ray   A type of electromagnetic radiation characterized by wavelengths of 100 angstroms or less.

X-Ray Beam   The radiation emerging from an x-ray generator or source.

X-Ray Spectrum   A portion of the electromagnetic spectrum with photon energies greater than 100 eV.

X-Ray Tube   An electronic tube in which x rays are generated.

Coolidge tube: A vacuum tube in which x rays are generated when the target (integral with the anode) is bombarded by electrons emitted from a heated filament and accelerated toward the anode across a high potential difference.

Crookes' tube: A vacuum discharge tube developed by Sir William Crookes in early experimental work with cathode rays. Wilhelm Roentgen first discovered that, in addition to the production of cathode rays, x rays were emitted during the operation of these tubes.

Gas tube: An early type of x-ray tube in which electrons were derived from residual gases within the tube.

Answers to Study Questions

Chapter 1

1. B. The embossed dot should always be toward the source, no matter which films you are doing.
2. D.
3. C. The film and the tooth should be parallel to each other, so both are perpendicular to the central ray.
4. B. Caries detection is primary, followed by crestal bone level detection.
5. B.
6. E.
7. A. Both maxillary and mandibular incisors and canines.
8. B. The mandibular canine is more anterior than the maxillary canine. Therefore, if the radiograph shows the distal half of the mandibular canine, it will almost always include all of the appropriate contacts.
9. B. Although answer A seems logical, it does not consider the potential for backscatter (secondary radiation that bounces off the patient and scatters almost straight backward toward you).
10. D. All will reduce radiation to the patient: A and B by reducing the exposure per film, and C by reducing the frequency of exposure.
11. B. You have to get an open view of the contact between the canines and premolars on this film because it often is not possible on the canine film.
12. D.
13. D.
14. D.

Chapter 2

1. A.
2. D.
3. B.
4. A.
5. A.
6. B.
7. A. The film mount should be opaque so as to transmit *no* light.
8. B. Never increase exposure times to make up for poor processing. If you checked the temperature, the time selected to develop should be accurate. The only alternative is weak chemicals that need to be changed.
9. C. Light from somewhere is causing the outline of the coin to show up.
10. B.
11. E. All of these will lead to fogging.
12. B. Answer C is incorrect, because even though the rinse between developing and fixing is eliminated with automatic processors, this does not significantly save time.
13. C.
14. B.
15. C.

Chapter 3

1. D. X rays have no mass and no density. They are pure energy.
2. C.

3. D.
4. B.
5. C.
6. D.
7. A.
8. A. We use such small amounts of electricity in x-ray production that we measure in milliamperes.
9. C. The kilovoltage makes the anode positive. Electrons (the ones hanging around the filament in a cloud) have a negative charge. When you push the exposure button, you are letting electrical current into the anode side, which makes it positive. The stronger the current (the more kilovoltage), the stronger the positive charge is on the anode. The stronger the current, the greater the attraction between the negative and positive sides of the x-ray tube.
10. A. Milliamperage has a direct effect on amount. Kilovoltage has a slight indirect effect.
11. D.
12. A.
13. D.
14. B. Although x rays are the desired end product, unfortunately heat is the primary product of x-ray generation.

Chapter 4

1. B. Although the word "high" may make one think in terms of "many," that is not the correct interpretation. If you had many shades of gray, there would be very little difference, or contrast, between each shade. If you had only black and white, there would be a lot of difference, or contrast, between the two shades.
2. D.
3. C.
4. E.
5. D.
6. D.
7. B. 10 mA $\times$ 30 impulses = 15 mA $\times$ 20 impulses.
8. D.
9. A. Rule of thumb: if you increase the kilovoltage by about 15, you double the density. Therefore, you need to cut the time in half.
10. D. To go from 16 inches to 4 inches, you divide by 4. If you square 4 (i.e., 4 $\times$ 4), you get 16. Dividing 60 by 16 gives you approximately 4 impulses.
11. D. Both decreasing the distance and increasing the milliamperage will reduce the time the most.
12. B. Use the rule in the answer for Question 9.
13. C. You divided the distance by 2. Now square it (i.e., 2 $\times$ 2 = 4), and divide the time (60 impulses) by 4 to get 15.
14. A. 10 mA $\times$ 60 impulses = 15 mA $\times$ 40 impulses.

Chapter 5

1. C.
2. B.

3. C. This is the only factor that is likely to change so drastically in so short a time.
4. A. Developer is the only alternative given that will make the films black.
5. B.
6. C.
7. E.

Chapter 6

1. D. The 68-year-old patient is the only one with enough teeth that would need that many films.
2. D.
3. B.
4. A.
5. E.
6. A.
7. B.
8. A.
9. C.
10. C.
11. B.
12. B.

Chapter 7

1. E. All of these.
2. A.
3. C.
4. D.
5. D.

Chapter 8

1. A
2. A.
3. B.
4. D.
5. C.
6. D.
7. B.

Chapter 9

1. A.
2. D.
3. B.
4. D.
5. A.
6. C.
7. A.
8. D.
9. C.

Chapter 10

1. C.
2. A, B, C.
3. A.
4. A.
5. F. All of these.

Chapter 11

1. C.
2. D.
3. C.
4. B.

Chapter 12

1. E.
2. D.
3. C.
4. C.
5. A.
6. D.
7. D.
8. B.
9. C.
10. C.

Chapter 13

1. D.
2. D.
3. B.
4. C.
5. A.
6. E.
7. D.
8. B.
9. A.
10. B.
11. B.
12. B.
13. E.
14. E.

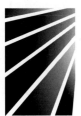

Index

Note: Page numbers in *italics* refer to illustrations; page numbers followed by t refer to tables.